SpringerBriefs in Cell Biology

A.M. Dygai • V.V. Zhdanov

Theory of Hematopoiesis Control

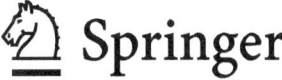 Springer

A.M. Dygai
Institute of Pharmacology
Russian Academy of Medical Sciences
Tomsk
Russia

V.V. Zhdanov
Institute of Pharmacology
Russian Academy of Medical Sciences
Tomsk
Russia

ISBN 978-3-319-08583-8   ISBN 978-3-319-08584-5   (eBook)
DOI 10.1007/978-3-319-08584-5
Springer Cham Heidelberg New York Dordrecht London

Library of Congress Control Number: 2014948745

Printed on acid-free paper

Springer is part of Springer Science+Business Media (www.springer.com)

Introduction

The accumulated data on the work of blood systems in norm and pathology showed that during balanced hematopoiesis, the neuroendocrine substances produce no direct action on proliferation and differentiation of hemopoietic cells. Under these conditions, the blood system demonstrates autonomic behavior controlled mostly by local mechanisms. In contrast, the leading role in upregulating hematopoiesis under extreme (stressful) conditions counterbalanced by the development of compensatory processes within the blood system is given to neuroendocrine regulatory structures.

At present, numerous regularities in the work of hemopoietic tissue as an integral system adequately reacting to varying conditions of external and internal environments are not evident. In the study of this problem during more than 30 years, we employed various experimental models of pathological processes (immobilization stress, acute and chronic blood loss, infectious inflammation, cytostatic and radiation myelosuppressions, encephalopathies of diverse genesis, experimental neuroses, spontaneous leucosis, *etc.*)

The results of these and other studies carried out by numerous workers had been described in a number of monographs published in our and other countries. They focused on specific problems relating to the control of hemopoiesis in norm and during the development of diverse pathologies. With deeper insight into this field and establishing new data widely discussed in literature (first of all, data on the hematopoietic stem cells and the regulatory molecules), we revisited the studies with previously employed models of pathological processes under a reliable methodology implying the study of the reactions of all major compartments of hematopoietic tissue to the action of a pathogenic factor with simultaneous testing of the functional activity of diverse regulatory systems. Without such a systemic approach, it is little probable to develop the theory of hematopoiesis control, whose numerous aspects we discussed many a time in previously published research papers and monographs. The authors are well aware of the fact that they cannot put the "final touch" to the problem of hematopoiesis since the study of any biological process seems to have no winning post.

However, a huge amount of accumulated data needs generalization and analysis to formulate the cornerstones of the theory of hematopoiesis control describing the regularities in the work of major subdivisions of hematopoietic tissue under normal and pathological conditions with due attention to interlacing activity of local and long-ranged regulatory systems.

The authors are grateful to the colleagues in State Research Institute of Pharmacology of Siberian Department of Russian Academy of Medical Sciences and in other agencies for courteously provided data.

Contents

Abbreviations

ANS	Autonomic nervous system
BFU-E	Burst-forming unit-erythroid
CFU-E	Colony forming unit-erythrocyte
CFU-F	Colony forming unit-fibroblast
CFU-G	Colony-forming unit–granulocyte
CFU-GEMM	Colony forming unit-granulocyte-erythrocyte-macrophage-megakaryocyte
CFU-GM	Colony forming unit-granulocyte macrophage
CFU-MM	Colony forming unit-monocyte macrophage
CFU-S	Colony-forming unit–spleen
CNS	Central nervous system
CSA	Colony-stimulating activity
EP	Erythropoietin
EPA	Erythropoietic activity
Flt3(Flk-2)-ligand	A member of cytokine moiety still not comprehensively characterized
GAGs	Glycosaminoglycans
G-CSF	Granulocyte colony-stimulating factor
GM-CSF	Granulocyte-macrophage colony-stimulating factor
HI	Hematopoietic islet
HIM	Hemopoiesis-inducing microenvironment
HSC	Hematopoietic stem cell
IFN-γ	Interferon γ
LPS	Lipopolysaccharide
MAF	Macrophage activating factor
M-CSF	Macrophage colony-stimulating factor
MPS	Mononuclear phagocyte system
MTD	Maximum tolerated dose
PHSC	Pluripotent hematopoietic stem cell
SCF	Stem cell factor (Steel factor)
SDF-1	Stromal cell-derived (chemotactic) factor

TGF-α (β)	Transforming growth factor α (β)
TNF-α(β)	Tumor necrosis factor α (β)
VEGF	Vascular endothelial growth factor
VG	Vegetative ganglia
VLA-5	Integrin ('very late antigen-5' = receptor for fibronectin)

Chapter 1
Mechanisms of Hematopoiesis Control

The blood system is composed of hematopoietic and hemolytic organs, circulating blood, and the control apparatus, which plays the important role in hematopoiesis by a balanced production of spectacular moiety of the cellular elements.

During a long period of time, the experimental and clinical data accumulated, which attested to the regulatory function of central nervous system (CNS) on the hemopoietic processes [16, 23, 25, 294]. Diverse external and internal stimuli generated in the receptive fields are processes by CNS with reflex action on the organs sustaining the required blood composition [188].

Transformation of nerve impulses into neurosecretory and humoral influences onto the blood system is performed predominantly in hypothalamo-hypophyseal complex. Stimulation of ventromedial and mammillary hypothalamic nuclei in animals up-regulates erythrocytosis and reticulocytosis in the peripheral blood resulting in an increase in erythrocytic mass [264, 265, 294]. According to S. Halvorsen, oxygen tension affects the work of hypothalamus, which elevates the production of erythropoietin in bone marrow transmitting the signals via nerves and hypophyseal hormones [264, 265]. The regulatory effects of the hypothalamus are projected not only to erythron, but also to the cells in the mononuclear phagocyte system. D. B. Konar and S. K. Manchanda showed that lesion of posterior medial hypothalamic structures inhibited the functional activity of macrophages [291].

The most important part of the blood is immune system. At present, the development of immune response is firmly established to depend on the regulatory influences of dopamine and serotonin [64, 65, 107, 184]. Activation of the serotoninergic system inhibits both humoral and cellular immune response [64, 65, 106, 343] and abrogates the mitogen-stimulated proliferation of T-cells [339]. In contrast, stimulation of dopaminergic system (1) elevates the content of CD4+-T cells in bone marrow and enhances the mitogen-induced proliferative response of T-lymphocytes; (2) increases the number of splenic antibody-forming complexes and rosette-forming cells in animals, and (3) abrogates the stress-induced depression of immune response [65, 106, 363]. While the regulatory effect of the serotoninergic system is mediated via hypothalamus, hypophysis, and the

© Springer International Publishing Switzerland 2014
A.M. Dygai, V.V. Zhdanov, *Theory of Hematopoiesis Control*,
SpringerBriefs in Cell Biology 5, DOI 10.1007/978-3-319-08584-5_1

adrenal glands, the effects of dopaminergic system are exerted via hypothalamus, hypophysis, and thymus.

An important role in the control of hematopoiesis is given to autonomic nervous system (ANS). Under the optimal performance of organism, the effect of ANS on hematopoiesis is commonly viewed as mediated predominantly via the control of metabolism and oxygen consumption, production of erythropoietin, as well as via trophogenic influences on intracellular metabolic processes in hematopoietic and stromal elements of bone marrow, which in their turn, control the proliferative potential of the hemopoietic cells [78, 141, 198, 52, 40]. The role of ANS transmitters in the control of hematopoiesis becomes even greater when an organism is exposed to diverse extreme (stressful) factors [60, 62, 141, 239]. To illustrate, injection of norepinephrine to mice treated with carboplatin weakens the myelosuppressive effect of this cytostatic agent [311, 312], while introduction of norepinephrine to the cultured bone marrow cells inhibits proliferation of CFU-GM. These effects are prevented by αl-adrenergic agonist prazosin. These data open the way to affect hematopoiesis via αl-adrenergic receptors. Probably, activation of these receptors triggers synthesis of TNF-β which inhibits proliferation of the cells.

The development of hypoplasia of bone-marrow hematopoiesis provoked by injection of 5-fluorouracil to CBA mice is accompanied by release of catechol-amines from chromaffin tissue of the adrenal glands [53, 182]. Moreover, these are direct correlation between concentration of catecholamines in the adrenal glands and cellularity of various hematopoietic lineages. Injection of dihydro-ergotamine and propranolol 3–5 min prior to and 5 h after administration of 5-fluorouracil lessened the degree of hypoplastic state of bone marrow on post-injection days 3 and 6 due to diminished drop in the count of lymphoid cells, although these agents decelerated regeneration of hematopoiesis starting from day 7. In contrast, administration of adrenoblockers prior to secondary release of the catecholamines from the adrenals stimulated postcytostatic recovery of hemato-poiesis accompanied by accelerated increase of cellularity in neutrophilic and erythroid lineages of the bone marrow. Injections of pentamine to mice under the same protocol to block the ANS ganglia and to disturb the release of sympathetic and parasympathetic neurotransmitters modulated hematopoiesis (previously suppressed with an antimetabolite) in a way, which in many respects mimicked the effects of adrenergic antagonists [4, 53, 182].

The dependence of recovery rate of bone-marrow hemopoiesis on activity of the sympathoadrenal system was also demonstrated with cyclophosphane [4, 53]. Really, combined administration of cyclophosphane with gangliolytic, α- or β-adrenolytic agents induced more pronounced suppression of bone-marrow and peripheral blood cellularity in CBA mice in comparison with individual use of this cytostatic. However, the use of these agents on day 3 after injection of cyclo-phosphane elevated the content of neutrophilic granulocytes and erythrocaryocytes in the bone marrow. Prior to the period of regeneration of the bone-marrow erythropoiesis, there was accelerated restoration of the count of neutrophilic leuko-cytes in circulating blood accompanied with a decrease in the content of micronuclear erythrocytes.

Numerous studies dealt with the role of hormones of pituitary-adrenal axis in the control of hematopoiesis. They established that hyperproduction of corticotropin could be accompanied with erythrocytosis while down-regulation of hypophyseal activity resulted in anemia [26, 274]. In addition, corticotropin inhibited lymphopoiesis [210], up-regulated the medullar hemopoiesis mostly due to hyperproduction of neutrophils, and promoted maturation of the cells of myeloid lineage [26, 307].

In physiological concentrations, the glucocorticoids inhibit migration of hemato-poietic stem cells (HSC) [145, 150]. The effects of glucocorticoids on the blood cells are dose-dependent. At low doses, they stimulate proliferation and differentiation of erythronormoblasts [150, 225, 240, 341]. In contrast, the high doses of corticosteroids inhibit erythropoiesis [225, 247, 254]. Depending on the dose, the corticosteroid hormones can also activate or inhibit the expansion of CFU-GM [91, 252, 290, 332].

Of great importance in the control influences of glucocorticoids over the performance of hemopoietic progenitors is interaction of these hormones with T-lymphocytes [123]. The exogenous glucocorticoids provoke migration of T-cells into the bone marrow [3, 223, 237] during the period relating to stimulation of erythropoiesis. The action of glucocorticoids on proliferation and differentiation of hemopoietic cells under basal conditions is mediated predominantly via their effects on metabolism and vascular tone [187]. Extirpation of the adrenal glands produced no effect on the number of hemopoietic islands and the content of precursors of erythro- and granulocytopoiesis in the bone marrow; moreover, it did not significantly shift of the blood system indices in mice [183]. During the balanced hematopoiesis, the adrenal hormones can control secretion of hemopoietic growth factors by the nonadherent cell elements of the bone marrow [183]. The role of glucocorticoids in the control of hematopoietic activity is greatly enhanced under the effect of stressors of diverse etiology [78, 90, 91, 228, 295, 314, 316]. Under these conditions, the corticosteroid hormones exert their effect on hematopoiesis mostly via some mediators such as T-cells [34, 35, 40].

Some studies focus on the role of hypophyseal-adrenal axis in proliferation and differentiation of the hemopoietic cells during cytostatic myelosuppressions. Thus, administration of acetate-cortisone in mice treated with lethal dose of carbo-platin protected the progenitor cells of granulomonocytopoiesis in the bone marrow [347]. This effect is accompanied by deceleration of expansion of CFU-S and CFU-GM in hematopoietic tissue. This hormone greatly increases resistance of the granulocyte-macrophage precursor cells against platinum and ^{3}H-thymidine. Moreover, hydrocortisone ameliorates the damaging effect of cytosine arabinoside to the blastoid cells during DNA synthesis performed in these cells [373].

In mice, the corticosteroids dexamethasone and prednisone efficiently protected the hematopoietic precursors against the toxic effect of 5-fluorouracil used at the dose of 200 mg/kg [295]. The greatest degree of protection of the cells against the side effects of the antimetabolite was observed after 2–3 intraperitoneal injections of dexamethasone (7.5 mg/kg) performed in the period between hour 7 prior to and hour 3 after injection of 5-fluorouracil. The protective effect was manifested by an increase in the number of proliferation colony forming units, which survived in the bone marrow 3 days after administration of the cytostatic agent. The content of medullar progenitors and blood cells returned to initial levels pronouncedly quicker in comparison with the animals treated with cytostatic alone.

In mice, dexamethasone used at about physiological concentration suppressed the growth of the erythro- and granulocytopoiesis precursors of regenerating bone marrow *in vitro* on day 5 after injection of 5-fluorouracil at 50 % MTD. It is of importance that introduction of dexamethasone in myelocaryocyte culture during the period of maximum depression (postinjection day 3) elevated content of granulocyte, macrophage, and fibroblastoid precursors [183]. The authors concluded that the direct effect of dexamethasone *in vitro* is mostly determined by the functional state of the cells.

Similar to dexamethasone, other hormones exert pronounced effects on the blood system. Both thyrotropin and thyroxin (a hormone of thyroid gland) stimulate erythropoiesis, which explains enhanced erythrocytosis or anemia during thyrotoxicosis or myxedema, correspondingly [26, 202, 221]. The erythroid lineage of erythropoiesis is also activated by testosterone. The female sex hormones produce the opposite effect [226, 244, 340].

Thus, the neuroendocrine system plays the key role in the control of medullar hemopoiesis suppressed by cytostatic agents. In this performance, the sympathoadrenal and hypophyseal-adrenal systems work as the peripheral pathways used by the central neuroendocrine mechanisms to tune the blood system via the erythro- and granulomonocytopoiesis progenitor cells.

The fundamental feature of hematopoiesis is a huge rate of cell production. This peculiarity of hematopoiesis is coupled to the corresponding great death rate of the blood cells after their life duty: in a healthy individual, 20 billion platelets, ten billion erythrocytes, and five billion leukocytes die in an hour [15, 19, 112]. During various pathologies, an extra need for the hemopoietic cells mobilizes the entire blood system, which results in a massive consumption of the hemopoietic progenitors needed to compensate the loss of the cells in the hierarchy downstream of hematopoiesis [19, 90, 189]. Similar challenges met repeatedly in the life of any evolutionary developed species could deplete the pool of hemopoietic progenitor cells if they are enlisted in any response to such challenges by the 'feedback mechanism'. Thus, it can be logically expected the existence of specialized local mechanisms, which adequately tune hematopoiesis at the level of committed and partially unipotential progenitors and limit the response of pluripotent hematopoietic stem cells (PHSC) to the long-distant neural and hormonal stimuli. These mechanisms assume responsibility for balance between different hemopoietic lineages in relation to the organism requirements [37, 152]. The role of such local regulatory system is played by the complex of cellular, extracellular, and the humoral factors located in immediate proximity to the hemopoietic elements known as hemopoietic (hemopoiesis-inducing) microenvironment.

The concept of hemopoiesis-inducing microenvironment (HIM) was advanced in 1976 by D. Trentin to explain the ability of some parts of hemopoietic tissue to induce maturation of the early hemopoietic progenitors to certain direction [177]. For instance, transplantation of hemopoietic cells to irradiated mice induces formation of erythroid colonies in the splenic red pulp and the development of granulocyte colonies near splenic capsule, trabeculae, and emptied follicles. In contrast to the spleen, the bone marrow is characterized with predominance of granulocyte colonies [134, 177, 266]. According to the data obtained in recent years, this fact can be explained by 'homing' of the hemopoietic precursor cells that had been preliminary committed in some specific regions of hemopoietic tissue to develop in a certain direction [152, 189, 266, 371]. The term HIM is commonly used to draw attention to ability of individual elements of hematopoietic microenvironment to promote predominant development of the cell that belong to certain hemopoietic lineages.

Diverse stromal and parenchymatous cells in hematopoietic organs with their metabolites are involved in formation of HIM. The microenvironment structure can be subdivided into mobile components and the stromal elements, which are fixed in the certain regions of the hemopoietic organs to form their 'meshwork'. The mobile cellular HIM components are mostly composed of some subpopulations of T-lymphocytes and macrophages, while the stromal HIM elements consist of macrophages, adipocytes, endothelial cells, the parts of microcirculatory bed, the nerve fibers, and the fibroblasts producing the components of extracellular matrix [37, 135, 181, 217, 266, 359].

The thymic lymphocytes are multifunctional mobile elements that easily form the structural complexes with macrophages and the stromal mechanocytes. Due to this property and ability to secrete a number of cytokines, the above lymphoid population plays the key role in the development of HIM and in the control over the processes of migration, proliferation, and differentiation of the hemopoietic cells [44, 90, 350]. It is of importance that such control can be either positive or negative in dependence on subpopulation of T-cells and their functional status. Under balanced hematopoiesis, the lymphocytes produce a rather limited amount of signaling substances, which control hematopoiesis. However, when affected by the mitogens, antigenic stimulation, or some stimuli of other modality, they gain the ability to secrete the early-acting growth factors IL-3 and GM-CSF irrespective to their polarization. IL-3 activates proliferation of the progenitor cells at different stage of maturation ranging from PHSC that aroused from the resting (dormant) phase to the committed precursors of all myelopoietic lineages, while GM-CSF stimulates expansion of CFU-GEMM and their progeny [134, 152, 273, 336]. Moreover, T-lymphocytes that differentiated into Th2-cells can secrete some lineage-restricted factors such as IL-5, which controls the production of eosinophils [134, 320, 326, 327]. In addition, Th2-lymphocytes secrete interleukins (IL-4, IL-9, IL-13, IL-17) which possess virtually no intrinsic hemotropic activity but affect the hematopoietic cells synergistically with other hemopoietins [260, 111, 199, 231, 238, 298, 357]. Thus, the activated CD4+-T-cells produce IL-17, which needs the release of G-CSF and the presence of transmembrane form of SCF to exert its stimulating effect on granulocytopoiesis [351].

The recent years changed radically the views on the role of T-cells in bone marrow, which inhibit both immune response and hematopoietic activity. According to modern conceptions, the suppressing activity of T-lymphocytes and some other hematopoiesis-regulating elements is mostly determined by their functional state instead of a certain 'suppressive' phenotype. This suppressing activity can be mediated via the intermembrane contacts with the target cells or via release of some soluble factors by T-lymphocytes. The latter can be presented by TNF-β produced by Th-lymphocytes and TGF-β synthesized by Th2-cells [199, 238, 327].

The most important components of HIM are the cells of mononuclear phagocyte system (MPS) with medullary macrophages playing an especially pronounced role. The population of these cells is characterized with great phenotypic and functional heterogeneity based on transitory expression of the functional features during maturation of monocytes [98, 152, 330, 348]. The bone marrow MPS cells control hematopoiesis by releasing diverse cytokines, forming the intermembrane contacts with the hemopoietic cells, and by producing the specific components of extracellular matrix (EDa- and EDb-variants of fibronectin) which is a basic part of HIM.

During these processes, the direct cooperation with hematopoietic elements is realized via formation of hemopoietic islets (HI), which are the structural and functional units of the hemopoietic tissue where reproduction and maturation of the hemopoietic cells from the committed to mature forms take place. In erythroid HI, the centrally located macrophage is surrounded with one or several layers of the erythronormoblasts at various stages differentiation stages which form a kind of 'corona'. Within this structure, the concentration of biologically active substances secreted by macrophage to control erythropoiesis is far greater than that in adjacent tissue [78, 98, 209, 227]. The resident macrophages and monocytes can produce cytokines that stimulate proliferation of the family of erythroid precursors where the most important member is erythropoietin. The mature medullar mononuclear phagocytes can also produce GM-CSF, which primes the early erythroid progenitors and potentiates the specific effect of erythropoietin [78, 95, 134, 320]. In line with lineage-restricted hemopoietins (G-CSF and M-CSF) which are also secreted by macrophages, GM-CSF is involved in the control of granulo- and monocytopoiesis. In addition, macrophages control the development of the cells in these lineages while being situated in HI, although in this case, they play a minor role in comparison with the stromal mechanocytes. However, the latter are controlled by such most important monokines as IL-1, IL-6, and TNF. Moreover, these secreted agents can up-regulate their own release by macrophages [95, 186, 218]. IL-1 and IL-6 are also important co-factors in stimulation of proliferation and differentiation of the early hemopoietic progenitors by other cytokines (SCF, Flt 3-ligand, G-CSF, IL-11, and IL-12), while IL-6 and G-CSF can trigger transition of HSC from resting G_0 phase to the cell cycle [37, 134, 152, 320]. Production of cytokines is dramatically augmented during activation of mononuclear phagocytes by bacterial LPS, the products of erythrocyte destruction, and T-lymphocytes [37, 78, 134, 320, 377].

Some factors produced by the cells of monocytic/macrophage lineage (specifically, IL-1 and TNF-α) can not only stimulate, but also inhibit the hematopoietic processes in dependence on the state of the target cells [277, 366]. For example, the macrophage-originated prostaglandins E_1 and E_2 exert a direct inhibitory effect on hemopoietic precursors. Similarly, such cell-produced agents as MPS, TGF-α, and NO inhibit cell colony formation and induce apoptosis [78, 176, 276, 310]. This phenomenon explains inhibition of erythropoiesis when the content of monocytic/macrophage cells in bone marrow is rather high [98].

An important functional feature of HIM cells is their mutual interaction in the control of proliferation and differentiation of the hemopoietic cells. A striking example of dependence of the functional state of MPS elements on qualitative composition of lymphocytes is given by secretion activity in macrophages induced with differently polarized T-cells. At this, 'classical' activation of NO production in macrophages is stimulated by Th1 cytokines IFN-γ and IL-2. In contrast, inhibition of NO production in macrophages (in this case, they are considered as alternatively activated) is exerted by Th2 cytokines IL-4, IL-10, and IL-13 [361]. The functional polarization of macrophages is viewed as an operation-rational process responsible for their optimal functional state [315]. Thus, the balance between Th1 and Th2 cells with their cytokines can underlie the positive or negative effect of the macrophages on hematopoiesis.

The key role in the development of stroma in all hematopoietic organs is given to stromal mechanocytes exemplified by fibroblastoid and reticular cells. These heterogenic adherent cells are not capable for recirculation and phagocytosis under the normal conditions but they display more or less expressed positive reactions to lipids, acid and alkaline phosphatase, as well as and non-specific esterase [78, 181, 376]. Among the fibroblastoid progenitors, the stem cells with high proliferative potential and progressively committed precursors are distinguished by degree of maturation. The mesenchymal stem cells also known as pluripotent mesenchymal stromal cells can differentiate not only into stromal meshwork but also into osseous or chondral elements, tendon cells, adipocytes, and possibly into the cells of other types [38, 322]. Pronounced polymorphism of stromal mechanocytes results not only from the above reasons, but it also reflects their functional heterogeneity in respect to hematopoietic cells and to other HIM elements [20, 39, 78, 189, 259]. The studies of composition of the bone marrow fibroblasts in humans revealed that the cells with long processes produce mechanical scaffold for the hemopoietic elements and make the solid basement of sinuses. They are also the major workshop to produce the extracellular matrix, which forms the microenvironment in the inner spaces of the bone marrow [151, 259]. Other type of the reticular cells with delicate processes form the close contacts with the young hemopoietic cells, which some authors consider as indication to functional interconnections [151]. Probably, these cells are the major producers of granulocyte and mixed HI in medullar tissue [78, 227]. It should be stressed that the cell clusters containing a fibroblastoid-like reticular cell and a macrophage typically incorporate the efferent nerve terminals [135, 286]. Based on this fact, Y. Kazuto and D. Terence advanced a novel anatomical unit, the 'neuroreticular complex' [286].

Similar to other cells in HIM, the stromal elements produce under the basal conditions a very limited and hard-to-detect amount of hematopoietically active substances [37, 39]. However, after stimulation with some cytokines (IL-1, IL-6, TNF) or due to interaction with activated macrophages and T-lymphocytes, the fibroblasts produce the early-acting growth factors and lineage-restricted hemopoietins. The early-acting factors comprise the stem cell factor (Steel factor, SCF), IL-11, and GM-CSF. SCF is one of two hemopoietic growth factors stimulating the specific receptors in stem cells and possessing tyrosine kinase-like activity. This cytokine is synthesized in two forms: one is bound to the cell surface, while other form is soluble. The bound SCF forms a protein locus on the surface of stromal cell, which binds to c-kit receptors available on HSC surface. Due to this interaction, HSC can glue to the stromal cells. The genetic defect of s1-locus of chromosome 10 coding SCF in mice dramatically degrades the ability of bone marrow stroma in mutant mice to glue HSC and potentiate their proliferation and differentiation in the presence of growth factors. SCF can induce division of PHSC dormant in G_0 phase. The combination of SCF, IL-6 (also secreted by the stromal cells) and/or IL-3 is the most potent stimulator for differentiation of these cells into the committed progenitors leading to production of blood cells. The activating effect of SCF spreads over the processes of proliferation and differentiation of the hemopoietic precursors of all maturation degree ranging from PHSC to unipotent cells [98, 134, 284, 318]. When added to cell culture with hemopoietic elements, IL-11 (a cytokine, produced by bone marrow stromal cells) sustains the growth of a small number of granulocyte-macrophage, multilineage, and blastoid colonies. However, when used in combination with IL-3 or SCF, IL-11 enhances colony formation. The synergistic effect of this cytokine with the early-acting hemopoietins is similar to that of IL-6. Both interleukins affect similarly G0 phase of the cell cycle of the early hematopoietic progenitors by shortening it and 'prompting' the stem cells to proliferation and differentiation [134, 287, 328]. The characteristic effects of IL-11 injected *in vivo* are stimulation of megacaryocytopoiesis, elevation of the count of the mature platelets in peripheral blood, and adipopenia in the experimental animals [253]. Inhibition of adipogenesis in line with stimulation of myelo- and lymphopoiesis are also observed during action of IL-11 in the long-term bone marrow culture [287].

The fibroblast-derived and late-acting hematopoietic growth factors are exemplified by G-SCF which controls the development of granulocytes from the committed to mature forms, and M-CSF that stimulates expansion of monocytic and macrophagal colonies and functional activity of the mature cells in MPS [37, 70, 78, 134, 220]. The neutrophil-activating factor IL-8 and IL-7, which stimulates maturation of the early hematopoietic progenitors in combination with IL-11 and Flt3-ligand, can be considered as the stromal cell-produced cytokines involved in the control of hematopoiesis [134, 345].

The adipocytes are also the key players in hematopoietic microenvironment. In the bone marrow, they are given several roles: while some of them just passively occupy the excess space in the medullar cavity, other cells are (1) active participants in systemic lipid metabolism, (2) local energy reservoirs in the bone marrow, (3) direct regulators of hematopoiesis, and (4) osteogenesis modulators [245, 378]. The role of adipocytes in the control of hematopoiesis is clearly demonstrated in various *in vitro* systems such as a long-term bone marrow culture known to be rapidly depleted without these cells [337]. While taking a part in forming the scaffold for the parenchymatous elements, these cells secrete some types of colony-stimulating factors. When stimulated with LPS or phorbol-2-myristate-13-acetate, the adipocytes can produce SCF and IL-6 [217, 337]. Moreover, some specific agents secreted by adipocytes affect proliferation and differentiation of the hematopoietic elements. For instance, hormone leptin stimulates bone marrow hematopoiesis (differentiation of granulocytes from the corresponding progenitors) and enhances the count of CD34+-cells in the peripheral blood. It is believed that leptin is involved in the development of leukocytosis related to obesity [289, 297]. At the same time, adiponectin (another product of adipocytes) selectively inhibits B-lymphopoiesis due to activation of cyclooxygenase and induction of synthesis of prostaglandins by HIM cells, which in their turn down-regulate the early types of B-lymphocyte progenitors but not the cell of other hemopoietic lineages [375]. However, a decrease in the number of adipocytes in hematopoietic tissue is characteristic of some myeloproliferative diseases [317]. The population of bone marrow adipocytes is reciprocally related to some other HIM elements such as osteoblasts, which is explained by their common origin from the mesenchymal stem cells. As a result, activation of adipogenesis is usually accompanied with inhibition of formation of the osseous tissue and vice versa, stimulation of osteogenesis inhibits formation of the adipose tissue [246, 322].

Of great importance is the role of such indispensable elements of bone marrow stroma as endotheliocytes. They serve the trophic and support functions, affect migration of bone marrow cells and take a part in the development of HI (predominantly of granulocyte and mixed type) [90, 151, 217]. Eventually, an alternative concept on the structural and functional organization of the bone marrow related to the vascular system became widely spread. According to this view, the primary structural role of the bone marrow is given to the hemopoietic cord with centrally situated arteriole encompassed and interwound with sinuses [197, 329]. Here the granulopoietic cells are distributed mostly along the wall of the central arteriole. The erythropoietic cells, located mainly around the sinus wall, form a continuous network of cords instead of separate islands. The megakaryocytes are positioned in close vicinity to the sinus wall at the extralumenal surface of sinus endothelium [329].

The spectrum of cytokines secreted by endotheliocytes is rather wide. In addition to the factors affecting non-differentiated hemopoietic progenitors (SCF, GM-CSF, IL-6, IL-11, flk-2-ligand), the vascular elements secrete the lineage-specific G-CSF, M-CSF, and thrombopoietin as well as VEGF-A [134, 197, 217, 337, 344]. The latter is also produced by immature hemopoietic progenitors being one of the most important regulators not only in vasculogenesis but also in hematopoiesis playing the certain role in providing HSC survivability. Moreover, endotheliocytes can produce the inhibitors of certain hemopoietic regulators such as macrophage inflammatory protein-2, TGF-β, and thymosin β-4 [197, 304]. Type IV and V collagen as well as laminins involved in formation of extracellular matrix are also the products of endotheliocytes [39, 98, 371].

Involvement of endothelial elements into the processes of migration of both mature and low-differentiated hemopoietic cells is effected via regulation of entry of the nucleated cells into circulation followed by their homing in the specific regions of hemopoietic tissue. Only a small part of hemopoietic progenitors leave the bone marrow spontaneously. This process engages the adhesive molecules of β-integrins and the corresponding ligands of the endotheliocytes [197, 324]. A rather low level of spontaneous migration implies that in addition to the adhesive molecules mediating the direct cell-cell contacts, the paracrine mechanisms play important role in migration of the cells into peripheral blood. Specifically, the studies revealed a great importance of VEGF-A, SDF-1 (a chemokine produced by stromal cells), G-CSF and other cytokines in involvement of endothelial cells in mobilization and homing of the hemopoietic progenitor cells [158, 197, 344].

The postnatal hematopoiesis takes place almost exclusively in bone marrow at the surface of endosteum or near it. This fact in company with the data on close contacts of the hemopoietic cells with osteoblasts reasoned to consider the latter to be active HIM components [151, 283, 379]. Many of the above cytokines and adhesion factors known to be important for normal hemopoiesis are produced by the osteoblasts. In addition, the bone marrow cells produce other proteins such as angiopoietin-1 and osteopontin, which not only can stimulate but also inhibit proliferation and differentiation of HSC. Some HSC (at least mostly immovable cells with low intensity of apoptosis and bound to osteoblasts) express tyrosine kinase receptor Tie2. *In vitro* interaction of Tie2 with its ligand angiopoietin-1 induces formation of the 'cobble-stone'- like areas, while *in vivo* it maintains the long-term repopulation activity of HSC. In addition, angiopoietin-1 restricts motility of HSC and induces their adhesion to the bone to protect the compartment with HSC from myelosuppressive stress [203, 204]. Osteopontin (according to D. N. Haylock, it is 'a bridge between osseous and hematopoietic tissues') is an acid glycoprotein, which similarly to angiopoietin relates to hematopoiesis as a factor that limits proliferation of the early hemopoietic progenitors. Thus, recent data attest to the key role of the osteoblasts and their products in maintaining the long-term repopulation activity of HSC, providing their immobile anchorage, protecting HSC against myelosuppressive stress, and limiting proliferation of the early hemopoietic progenitors [204, 269, 270]. At the same time, the cells of osseous tissue are controlled by some hemopoietic elements. For instance, megakaryocytes *in vitro* can stimulate proliferation and differentiation of osteoblasts, as well as inhibit the formation of osteoclasts [283]. Similar to endotheliocytes, the osteoblasts play an important role in homing the normal hemopoietic progenitors and the leukemic cells, which in the latter case leads to formation of so-called leukemic niche [331].

The principle role in the control of functional activity of the hemopoietic cells is played by adhesive properties of microenvironment elements. The intermembrane binding (gluing) promote (1) transmission of the regulatory information and signaling molecules, (2) migration of the progenitor cells followed by their homing in the specific regions of hemopoietic tissue, and (3) exposure of the hematopoietic growth factors in biologically available forms [135, 266, 371]. The leading role in association of the hemopoietic and stromal cells is played by membrane-bound class of regulators comprising the family of surface adhesion molecules (integrins and selectins) as well as type II histocompatibility antigens [290, 302, 371]. Some data indicate alterations in association bonds between the hematopoietic cells and the microenvironment elements during various hematological diseases [256, 317], which probably play a significant role in their pathogenesis.

As we mentioned before, HIM elements exert their effects on hematopoiesis not only by producing the hemopoietic activities. The stromal cells and specialized macrophages produce collagen, the reticulin fibers, fibronectin, laminin, tenascin, hemonectin, and some other components of the filamentous network of extracellular matrix, as well as proteoglycans and glycosaminoglycans (GAGs), which are the cornerstone components of the connective tissue [78, 98, 157, 259].

The extracellular substance of hematopoietic tissue includes collagen of five types: the type I, II, and III collagens are secreted by fibroblasts, while type IV collagen (a protein of basal membrane) and type V collagen are produced by endotheliocytes. Collagen plays the key role among the proteins in extracellular matrix by providing its mechanical stability. Activation of collagen synthesis in the bone marrow up-regulates production of the hemopoietic progenitors, while its inhibition suppresses this production [98, 213].

Fibronectin is a heterodimeric glycoprotein with disulfide bonds at the carboxyl terminus. This molecule has several functional sites mediating adhesion of the host cell to collagen and laminin. It is believed that fibronectin serves the anchorage function towards the hemopoietic precursors committed to the development in erythroid direction [95, 367].

Laminin is a glycoprotein composed of three intersecting protein chains, which form a tertiary structure stabilized with disulfide bonds. This major adhesive protein is secreted by endotheliocytes to become a part of basal membrane [261, 335].

Hemonectin is a protein found only in the bone marrow. It is hypothesized that this protein predominantly binds to the immature granulocytes regulating their release from the bone marrow as they mature [219].

In addition to fibrous structures, the extracellular matrix comprises so-called 'ground substance' with glycosaminoglycans (GAG), the linear polymers composed of disaccharide repeat units that form proteoglycans by binding to a protein. GAG molecule necessarily incorporates either glycosamine or galactosamine residues. The second monomer is represented by D-glucuronic or L-iduronic acids. According to the content of hexosamines (either greater or smaller than 4 %), GAGs are conventionally subdivided into acid and neutral ones [8, 157].

The major GAGs in the connective tissue are hyaluronic acid (40 % of all GAG in bone marrow), chondroitin-4-sulfate, chondroitin-6-sulfate, heparan sulfate, heparin, dermatan sulfate, and keratan sulfate [8, 358]. The presence of GAGs as indispensable elements in the cell surface or granular structures, their pronounced polyanionic properties, and the peculiarities of their conformation promoting interaction with the proteins to modify the biological activity of the affected proteins, attest to the fact that GAGs are involved into direct cell-cell interactions. GAGs activate mitoses of the early erythroid and granulocyte progenitor cells; moreover, they down-regulate differentiation of granulocyte progenitors [95, 135]. According to some authors, effect of GAG is mediated by increasing membrane permeability of hemopoietic cells to calcium followed by activation of the cyclic nucleotide system resulting in elevation of cAMP concentration. Thus, GAGs up-regulate production of the second messengers, which mediate a rapid spread of the signal from the receptors in hemopoietic cells to their genome under the control of the corresponding cytokines [98, 355].

According to modern views, a GAG complex with the above extracellular proteins is considered as a structure that sustains a certain level of the hemopoietic growth factors and modulates their functions. The extracellularly polymerized proteins, polysaccharides, and proteoglycans bind the cytokines and present them in an accessible form to the receptors localized on the surface of the hemopoietic progenitors [135, 217, 359]. The complexes formed by cytokines and extracellular matrix components are characterized with greater affinity to the specific receptors than cytokines *per se*. In their turn, receptors of the corresponding growth factors stimulate dissociation of GAG-cytokine complexes. Various components of extracellular matrix also incorporate the adhesive molecules, whose expression rate is controlled by hemopoietic growth factors IL-3, GM-CSF, and SCF [302, 359, 371]. It is of importance that the surface of most cells in the bone marrow incorporates the receptors for proteins of the extracellular matrix. These receptors known as integrins are taxonomized as a special receptor group, which includes in particular, the proteins mediating cell binding to certain components of the extracellular substance. For instance, integrin VLA-5 of hemopoietic cells is the receptor for fibronectin. Interaction of integrins with their ligands affects (1) production of second messengers in the hemopoietic cells, (2) the cytoskeleton parameters, (3) the number of receptors on the plasmatic membrane, (4) cytokine secretion, (5) function of ribosomes, and (6) transcription of genes in these cells [95, 372]. Taking into consideration that many cytokines control synthesis of the components of extracellular substance and can remodel it, the mutual relations between humoral factors and extracellular matrix of HIM becomes evident [359, 371]. Thus, the ground substance in the connective tissue is a very active medium, which can be therefore considered as the most important regulator of hematopoiesis.

The local and long-distant control systems of hematopoiesis are characterized with redundancy of the regulator influences yielding very precise tuning of overall hemopoietic process (Fig. 1.1). Specific organization of HIM helps its structures to efficiently modulate the instructive signals of macroorganism directed to the hematopoietic tissue. In this performance, HIM can completely protect some hemopoietic elements from the influence of these signals while modulating and channel them to other hemopoietic structures. HIM plays this role by engaging the direct cell-cell contacts with hematopoietic elements and by secreting the hemopoietic growth factors.

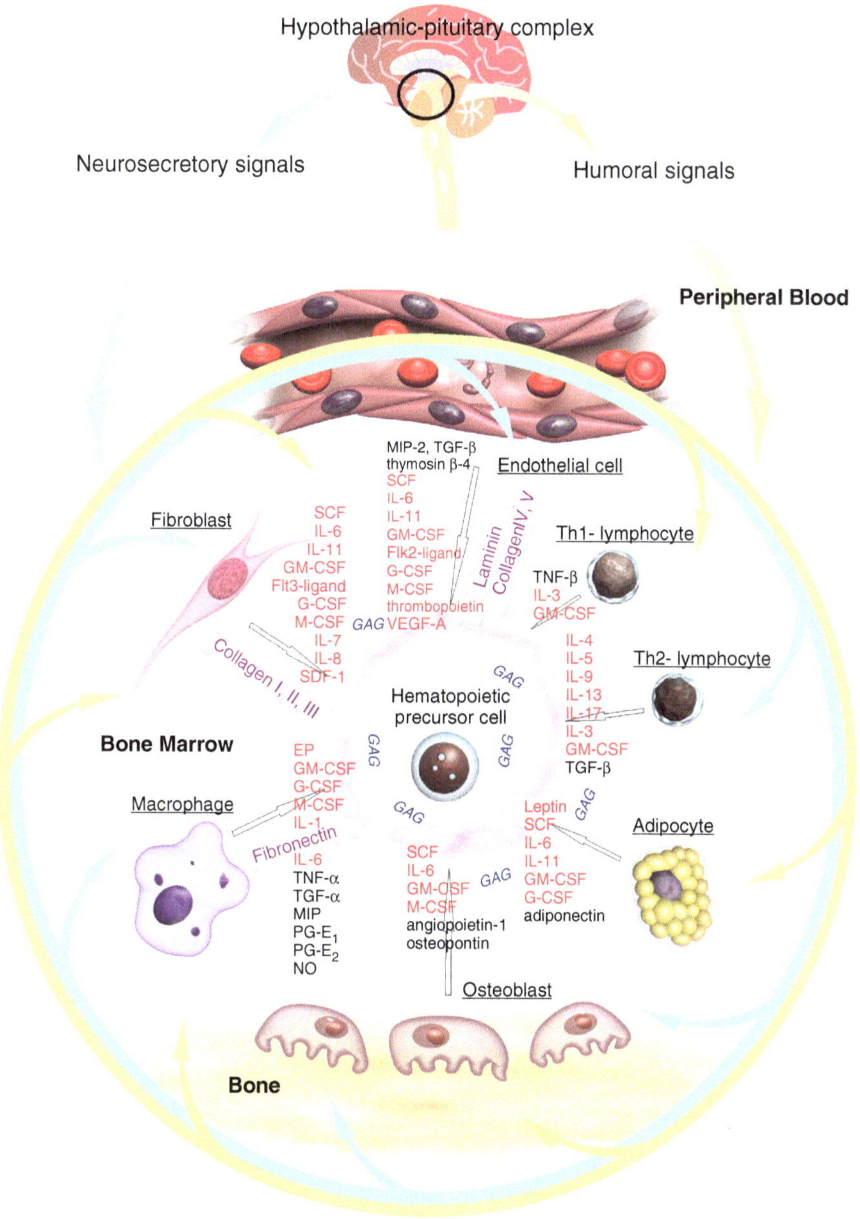

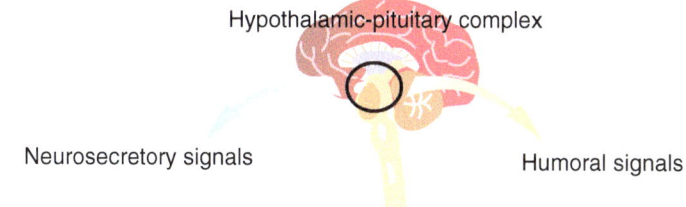

Hypothalamic-pituitary complex

Neurosecretory signals   Humoral signals

Peripheral Blood

MIP-2, TGF-β
thymosin β-4   Endothelial cell
SCF
IL-6
Fibroblast   SCF   IL-11
SCF   GM-CSF   Th1- lymphocyte
IL-6   Flk2-ligand
IL-11   G-CSF   TNF-β
GM-CSF   M-CSF   IL-3
Flt3-ligand thrombopoietin   GM-CSF
G-CSF   *GAG* VEGF-A
M-CSF
IL-7   IL-4
IL-8   IL-5   Th2- lymphocyte
SDF-1   IL-9
Collagen I, II, III   IL-13
GAG   IL-17
Hematopoietic   IL-3
precursor cell   GM-CSF
Bone Marrow   TGF-β
EP
GM-CSF
G-CSF
Macrophage   M-CSF
IL-1   Leptin   Adipocyte
Fibronectin   IL-6   SCF
TNF-α   SCF   IL-6
TGF-α   IL-6   IL-11
MIP   GM-CSF *GAG* GM-CSF
PG-E₁   M-CSF   G-CSF
PG-E₂   angiopoietin-1 adiponectin
NO   osteopontin

Osteoblast

Bone

Fig. 1.1 Functional diagram of the long- and short-distance regulatory structures involved in the control of hematopoiesis

Chapter 2
Alterations in Blood System Induced By Extreme Conditions Provoking No Myelosuppression

Numerous data accumulated about various features of the performance of blood system in norm and pathology leave unresolved many a problem on the regularities in the mechanisms integrating the hematopoietic tissue into a sophisticated dynamic system, which adequately responds to the changing conditions in the internal and external environment. The overall solution to these problems cannot be reached without systemic approach [51, 181, 362].

In our studies carried out for many years, we employed diverse experimental models of the pathological processes (immobilization stress, acute and chronic blood loss, infectious inflammation, cytostatic and radial myelosuppressions, encephalopathies of different genesis, experimental neuroses, and spontaneous leucosis). These studies assessed the cell performance in basic subdivisions of the hematopoietic tissue and activity of the local and long-distant interacting regulator systems. Despite the fact that the alterations in the blood system and the underlying mechanisms triggered by pathogenic factors of different nature are mostly non-specific and typical, the particular reaction of the blood system is determined by the nature of the stimulus.

Numerous studies showed that the formation of general adaptation syndrome developed under the action of extreme (stressful) stimulants of diverse nature involves all the known homeostatic systems, the system of blood included. The early changes in hematopoiesis (the first stage of the stress reaction) appear during 12 h after the onset of stimulation and include (1) decrease in cellularity of the spleen and thymus due to enhanced migration and inhibition of lymphocytic proliferation [99, 100]; (2) the development of neutrophilic leukocytosis in the peripheral blood (resulting from mobilization of bone marrow reserve granulocytes and the marginated leukocyte pool); (3) eosinopenia; and (4) lymphopenia. The latter is related to migration of lymphoid cells from the peripheral cells to the bone marrow, lymph nodes, and various tissues [60, 61]. This migration results in the 'lymphoid peak' in the bone marrow caused by increasing content of T- and B-lymphocytes [59, 60]. The development of lymphocytosis in the bone marrow is accompanied by enhancement of its immune competence [100], activation of granulocytopoiesis

© Springer International Publishing Switzerland 2014
A.M. Dygai, V.V. Zhdanov, *Theory of Hematopoiesis Control*,
SpringerBriefs in Cell Biology 5, DOI 10.1007/978-3-319-08584-5_2

manifested by an increase in the number of immature forms of myeloid series [60] and CFU-S [100]. The second stage is characterized by the development of hyperplasia of myeloid tissue and the growth of individual hematopoietic lineages. At this period, the productive enhancement of splenic cellularity is observed together with continuing migration of the lymphocytes from the thymus. Only the long-term action of a stressor (14–16 days) leads to exhaustion of compensatory potencies of the hemopoietic tissue and inhibition of all hemopoietic lineages [60]. However, involvement of the HIM-forming elements in these reactions was little studied. Logically, in a series of experimental studies carried out in Department of Pathological Physiology and Experimental Therapy, we employed the model of immobilization stress to examine the role of neuroendocrine and cellular hemopoietic control mechanisms in the formation of the adaptive processes in the hemopoietic tissue.

We showed that during stress, ANS exerted direct (receptive) and indirect (mediated via HIM-factors) stimulating effect on the hemopoietic precursors (CFU-E, CFU-GM) resulting in hyperplasia of erythroid and granulocyte medullar lineages accompanied with an increase in cellularity of the peripheral blood [53]. The hemopoietic tissue of mice subjected to 6–10-h immobilization displayed activation of the stem and committed stromal cells responsible for HIM transfer observed during post-immobilization days 3–5 [41, 76] accompanied by an increase in the number of macrophage-positive and macrophage-negative HI (days 4–7) [28, 54, 190]. On days 5–6, the colony- and cluster-forming potency of the bone marrow enhanced [192, 55], while the number of myelocaryocytes increased (on days 6–7) mostly due to elevation in the content of cellular elements of erythroid and granulocyte hemopoietic lineages [77, 55, 81]. In the peripheral blood, reticulocytosis, erythrocytosis, neutrophilosis, and monocytosis developed on days 6–8 [32, 55, 90].

Thymectomy performed 1 month prior to immobilization prevented the described alterations in the medullar hematopoiesis in the stressed mice. There was neither bone marrow hyperplasia nor increase in the score of CFU-GM or CFU-E in the thymectomized mice [77, 192, 41]. Elimination of hemopoietic activation in mice that had been thymectomized 1 month prior to immobilization indicates that the regulator T-cells belong to the short-lived population of T-lymphocytes. Namely these cells are the first to be eliminated in an animal subjected to thymectomy [145]. However, the mere deficiency of T-lymphocytes not accompanied with additional damaging stimulation produced no significant effect on the state of medullar hemopoiesis [44, 192]. Probably, under the optimal conditions of life, the lymphocytes play a minor role in sustaining hemopoiesis.

After transplantation of 4×10^7 viable thymocytes to thymectomized stressed mice, the count of CFU-GM and CFU-E, the total number of myelocaryocytes as well as the number of morphologically differentiated erythroid or granulocyte elements virtually did not differ from the corresponding values of the sham-thymectomized mice. However, hyperplasia of medullar hemopoiesis did not develop in the mice grafted with thymus in a diffusion chamber. Similarly, stimulation of hematopoiesis was not observed during blockade of T-lymphocytic system with antithymocyte serum. Under the conditions of immobilization stress, T-cells project their regulating influences not only to committed hemopoietic precursor cells, but also to more adult and morphologically differentiated hematopoietic elements [81]. The experimental data attesting to abrogation of hematopoietic stimulation against the background intraperitoneal injection of specific antilymphocyte antibodies suggest that proliferation of the progenitor cells is initiated by the immature lymphocytes [27]. In the following, the consecutive changes of T-lymphocyte population accompany the development of hyperplasia of the medullar hemopoiesis: immature cells are dominant on day 4 after the onset of immobilization stress to be replaced by helper (day 6) and suppressor (day 8) T-cells.

Prior to rising total cellularity in the bone marrow of stressed mice, the total number of HI in their hematopoietic tissue significantly increased [55, 90, 190]. In the stressed animals injected with algal polysaccharide carrageenan, which selectively inhibits MPS but not the lymphocytes, blockade of macrophages completely abrogated enhancement in production of not only HI, but also the progenitor cells as well as the development of bone marrow hyperplasia observed in control animals on days 5–6 after immobilization. Similar disturbances developed in the hematopoietic tissue during adaptation syndrome in thymectomized mice with blocked MPS attest to the fact that the mechanisms employed by these systems to exert their regulator influences on hematopoiesis are closely related and interconnected. This is also corroborated by inhibition of stimulation of HI production in the bone marrow of the stressed mice after injection of the antithymocyte serum. In immobilized thymectomized mice with MPS blocked by carrageenan, the transplanted thymocytes lost the ability to stimulate production of HI, committed progenitors, and the morphologically differentiated hemopoietic cells. When the role of stromal microenvironment in the control of medullar hemopoiesis in the stressed animals was examined with the method of heterotopic transplantation [41, 76], it turned out that beginning on day 3 after immobilization, the bone marrow activated the stromal cells responsible for HIM transfer. This process enlisted not only the committed stromal elements forming the 'primary' heterotopic hemopoietic focus, but also the stem stromal elements constructing the 'secondary' hemopoietic focus. Thymectomy completely prevented the above alterations in the stressed animals.

The following studies of dynamics of cytokine production by the bone marrow in stressed mice revealed a dramatic enhancement of spontaneous production of IL-1 activity as early as on day 1 after onset of immobilization, thereupon this activity moderated but increased again on day 4 [33, 57]. In the next days, the potency of examined supernatants to stimulate proliferation of thymocytes decreased. Under stimulation of the adhering elements of the bone marrow with LPS, the maximal IL-1 activity was observed on experiment day 4, and this activity remained significantly enhanced on days 5–6. Up-regulation of production of IL-3 activity by non-adherent medullar nucleated cells was observed starting from day 1, and it attained maximum level on days 4–5 after stimulation. In the experiments where the non-adherent medullar nucleated cells were stimulated with concanavalin A, up-regulation of production of IL-3 activity was observed on days 1–2 after immobilization.

The study of colony-stimulating activity (CSA) of supernatants from murine bone marrow cells showed that the maximum values of CSA in the conditioned media harvested from adherent and non-adherent medullar nucleated cells were attained on days 4, 6 and days 2, 5, correspondingly. In experiments with LPS-stimulated adherent medullar cells, the maximum values of CSA were observed on days 3, 4, and 6, which surpassed the initial level by 6.7, 4.7, and 3.3 times, respectively. It should be noted that addition of concanavalin A produced virtually no effect on production of CAS by the medullar non-adherent nucleated cells. At the same time, pronounced elevation of macrophage-stimulating activity was revealed in the examined supernatants on day 3 after immobilization under incubation of the non-adherent medullar cells with concanavalin A.

Stressful conditions enhanced the production of erythropoietic activity (EPA) in the bone marrow mostly on account of the adherent cells. When the culture was supplemented with the mitogens, the ability to up-regulate the production of ery-throid colonies increased in the supernatants harvested both from the adherent and non-adherent medullar nucleated cells. The study of dynamics of TNF-activity showed that the maximum of its spontaneous production was attained on experi-ment day 3, and production was enhanced until day 5 after stimulation. In superna-tants harvested from LPS-stimulated adherent medullar cell elements, the maximum elevation of TNF-activity was observed on experiment day 5.

Analysis of the changes in dynamics of medullar synthesis of the regulator molecules in mice subjected to immobilization stress revealed two characteristic stages. The first stage was observed on days 1–2 after the onset of stressful stimulation, and it included induction of the cells capable to produce IL-1 and IL-3 activities, which probably culminated in stimulation of HSC proliferation. Specifically, IL-1 is known to enhance sensitivity of the stem cells to IL-3 and to affect HSC pool, prompting it to enter into the cell cycle [140]. However, just as the stem cells termi-nate G_0 phase of the cell cycle, their further proliferation needs the presence of IL-3 [301]. It is hypothesized that IL-1 activates T-lymphocytes that accumulate in the bone marrow during the first hours of the development of stress reaction [60]. During this period, the migrating T-cells produce IL-3 required to support HSC proliferation. At any case, the primary elevation of IL-3 activity in the bone marrow is paralleled with rising CFU-S content [60]. Probably, during the early terms of the development of stress reaction, IL-1 stimulates CSA production by the medullar nucleated cells.

An important role in the development of the stress-induced alterations is given to the neuroendocrine apparatus – specifically, to the hypothalamic-pituitary-adrenal axis [113]. Modeling the hypocorticoid state with bilateral adrenalectomy prevented the stress-induced accumulation of T-lymphocytes in hemopoietic tissue. Moreover, these models displayed no signs of the development of hyperplasia among the committed and morphologically differentiated myeloid elements [191].

The second stage in production of humoral biologically active factors is charac-terized with migration of hemopoietic regulator T-lymphocytes into the bone marrow of the stressed mice on experiment days 3–5, where they stimulate proliferation and differentiation of the progenitor cells of erythro- and granulomonocytopoiesis and their more differentiated descendants [81]. Proliferation of the progenitor cells is initiated by immature T-lymphocytes that exert their control effects in cooperation with macrophages and stromal elements of the bone marrow [55]. Probably, this population of lymphocytes takes a part in up-regulating synthesis of IL-3 and macrophage-activating factor on day 3 after the onset of stressful stimulation. The activated macrophages start to produce IL-1 and TNF, which in their turn, stimulate the medullar nucleated cells to synthesize the colony-stimulating activities leading to stimulation of proliferation and differentiation of the committed hemopoietic progenitor cells (Fig. 2.1).

To clarify the role of thymus in the control of cytokine production by the bone marrow cells in stressed mice, we carried out the experiments on thymectomized and sham-operated animals. The resulting data agree with those on migration of immature T-lymphocytes into the bone marrow starting from post-immobilization day 3 [67]. Probably, namely these elements are the major players in up-regulating IL-3 synthesis by the medullar cells in the stressed mice. However, even the thymectomized animals demonstrated enhancement of IL-3-like activity, although it was not so pronounced as in sham-operated mice. Seemingly, production of IL-3-like activity in the bone marrow can be mediated not only by T-lymphocytes, but also by other cells – specifically, by the progenitors of thymic lymphocytes [130]. The concerned experiments showed that elevation of CSA produced by non-adherent fraction of the medullar nucleated cells is also a thymus-depending process.

Of principal importance is influence of thymectomy on functional activity of the adherent cells in the bone marrow. Inadequate reaction of the adhering elements to stress-stimulated thymectomized animals is evident. Such animals demonstrated no pronounced increase in IL-1 activity on post-immobilization day 1. On the contrary, they enhanced CSA production. Probably, the control over IL-1 and TNF production is mediated via different mechanisms. While in the thymectomized mice up-regulation of IL-1 synthesis was not observed only on post-immobilization day 1, although the potency of the medullar adherent cells to produce IL-1 did not significantly differ from that in the sham-operated mice on post-immobilization days 3–8, the production of TNF-activity in the thymectomized mice did not increase after stressful stimulation. After supplementing the culture medium with stimulator (LPS), elevation of TNF-activity was not so much pronounced as in the sham-operated animals. Probably, thymectomy changes the initial level of functional activity of regulator cells in the bone marrow, which is indirectly attested by an enhanced level of CSA in the supernatants harvested from the adherent and non-adherent myelocaryocytes of unstressed thymectomized mice.

Thus, both early and the subsequent stress-induced alterations in HIM functional activity are controlled by the thymus. However, some populations of the adherent elements of HIM work independently on the thymus and probably namely these cells are involved in compensation of the changes observed in the hematopoietic system after thymectomy.

Numerous studies focused on the effects of acute stressful stimulation on an organism. However, far smaller number of works examined the effects of chronic or recurrent stressful stimulation. The bone marrow of mice subjected to multiple repeated 15-h immobilizations demonstrated dramatic suppression of erythro- and lymphopoiesis accompanied by the corresponding changes in the peripheral blood.

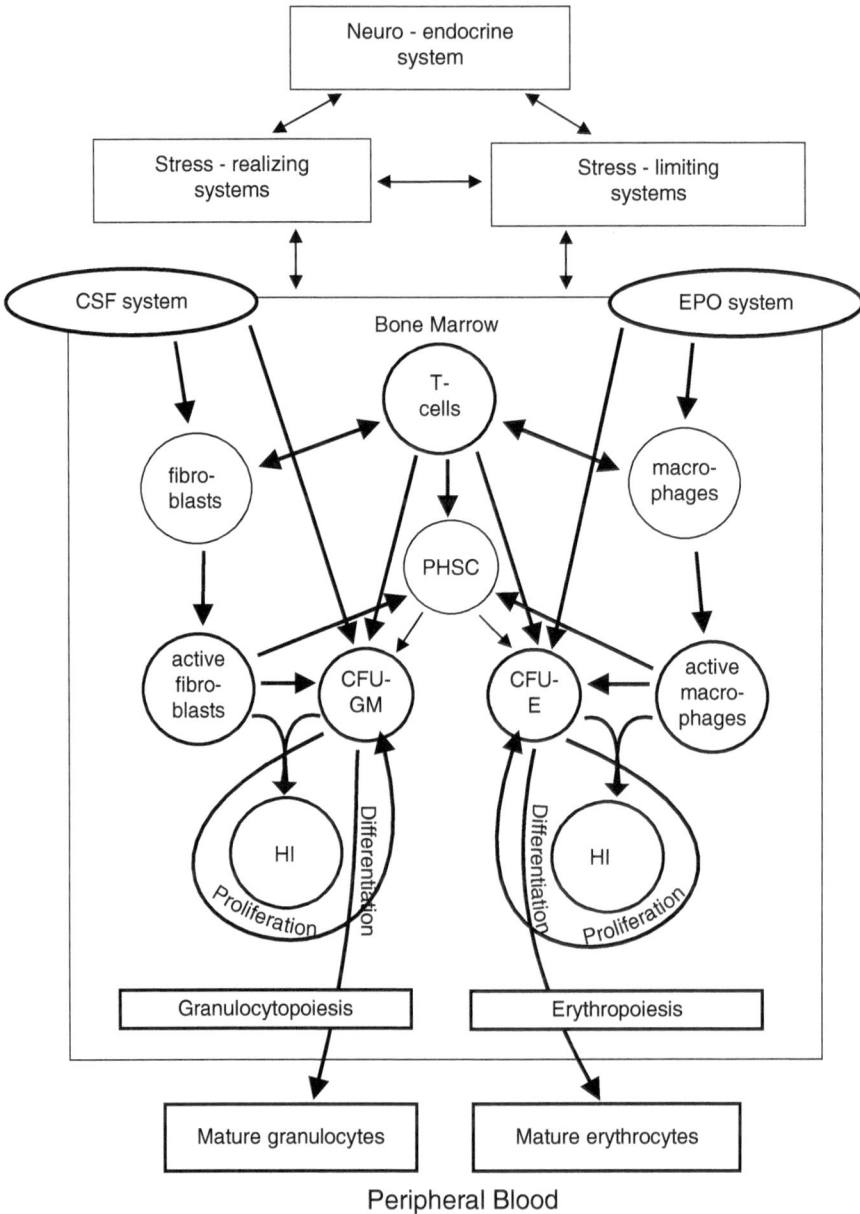

Fig. 2.1 Control of hematopoiesis during immobilization stress. The fine continuous lines correspond to negligible effect on the indicated structures, while the heavy lines represent activation

The early terms of such experiments were characterized with a drastic increase in the count of erythroid precursors by at least ten times relatively to the intact control. Increase in the medullar score of CFU-E was accompanied with up-regulation of EPA production by the non-adherent and adherent myelocaryocytes. There was a persistent increase in the level of EPA in the blood serum of the stressed animals, which could be related to the extramedullary production of erythropoietin [346]. A decrease in the score of erythrocaryocytes accompanied with insignificant rise in the number of erythroid islets and elevated production of erythroid precursors can be related to abnormalities in the processes of differention of the erythroid cells, since according to modern views, HI is the region where the hemopoietic cells maturate from the precursor stage to the mature forms [98, 227].

Enhancement of granulocyte-macrophage colony formation during multiple immobilization stimulation was also observed starting from experiment day 1 against the background decrease in the number of granulocyte HI in the bone marrow relatively to initial level. The multiple stressful stimulation elevated CSA score both in the conditioned media harvested from myelocaryocyte cultures and in the blood serum of the experimental animals.

Multiple 15-h immobilization resulted in pronounced involution of the thymus not accompanied by marked accumulation of Thy-1,2$^+$-cells in the bone marrow at the early terms of experiments, although immobilization stress dramatically increased the count of T-lymphocytes [90]. Thus, disturbance of T-cell migration into the bone marrow and their interaction with the resident macrophages and the stromal mechanocytes can explain the absence of hyperplasia of medullar hemopoiesis during multiple stressful stimulation. However, Thy-1,2$^+$-cells significantly accumulated in the bone marrow at later terms of experiment. Probably, this cell population is responsible for up-regulation of IL-3 synthesis in the supernatants harvested from the non-adherent bone marrow cells of the stressed mice. Enhancement of IL-1 production in the conditioned media of the adherent myelocaryocytes was observed starting from experiment day 1, and it was sustained to the end of the observation period, which is viewed as manifestation of some unspecific response of an organism to any damaging stimulation [334]. In its turn, elevated IL-1 stimulates the bone marrow cells to produce both EPA and CSA at the early stages of the stress experiments.

Thus, this lack of hyperplasia of medullar hemopoiesis observed despite enhanced production of the hematopoietic precursors and up-regulation of synthesis of the short-range hemopoietic regulators, as well as insignificant elevation in the number of HI attest to severe dysregulation of proliferation and differentiation of the hemopoietic cells under such powerful stimulation of an organism as the daily 15-h immobilization.

During acute inflammation (the peritonitis model), the abnormalities in the control over production of the white blood cells are predominant [79], which is explained by the key role of neutrophils, the must cells, and monocytes in the development and culmination of the inflammatory process [45, 78, 114, 251, 380].

Inflammation is accompanied by pronounced activation of bone marrow granulomonocytopoiesis. During inflammation, the changes in cellularity of the above hemopoietic lineages are phasic in character. The score of immature forms of medullar neutrophilic granulocytes grows and attains maximum on experiment days 3 and 6, the corresponding days for monocytes being 2 and 6 [78].

These changes in the bone marrow granulomonocytopoiesis are mostly paralleled by the dynamics of mature cells content in the peripheral blood. Really, the development of neutrophilic leukocytosis is characterized with maxima on experiment days 1 and 6. Enhancement of the blood monocytic score was also bi-phasic. Probably, the development of neutrophilic leukocytosis observed at the early period in the development of acute inflammation (experiment day 1) is underlain by re-distributive mechanisms as indicated by dramatic decrease in the score of mature forms of medullar neutrophilic granulocytes at this period (probably, due to their accelerated release into the peripheral blood). At later stages of the inflammatory process, the development of neutrophilosis and monocytosis is explained by up-regulation of the production of the corresponding forms of the cell elements, which is attested not only by spectacular increase of the count of immature granulocytes and monocytes in the bone marrow tissue, but also by pronounced elevation of the number of mature (rod and segmented nucleus) forms of the polymorphonuclear leukocytes whose score attained maximum to experiment day 6.

The development of bone marrow hyperplasia during inflammation is related to stimulation of proliferation and differentiation of the committed precursors of granulo- and monocytopoiesis whose medullar score varies in oscillating manner. Analysis of morphologic preparations of the mature colonies concluded that these events are accompanied with stimulation of release of three types of colony-forming units from the bone marrow: CFU-GM (granulocyte macrophage), CFU-G (granulocyte), and CFU-MM (monocyte macrophage). We are tempted to relate this phenomenon with biphasic increase of HI score in the hematopoietic tissue (predominantly, of granulocyte and mixed types). Really, the latter fact attests to HIM functional activation. During inflammation, the cell elements in hemopoietic microenvironment start to produce the short-range humoral factors, which stimulate the processes of proliferation and differentiation of the hemopoietic cells. As early as day 1 after introduction of inflammatory agent, production of IL-1 by the adherent nucleated cells was pronouncedly up-regulated. On experiment days 1, 2, and 8, the potency of macrophage-activating factor significantly increased in the conditioned media harvested from the non-adherent myelocaryocytes. Similarly, soon after the onset of observation period, elevation of CSA was established in the supernatants harvested from the adherent, non-adherent and medullar elements as well as in the blood serum, which indicates an important role of the colony-stimulating factors (probably including those produced by the leukocytes in the inflammatory focus) in the control of bone marrow granulomonocytopoiesis and in shaping the systemic response of the hematopoietic tissue during inflammation. However, both acute inflammation and other stress reactions are also accompanied with activation of erythropoiesis prompted by up-regulation of HIM functional activity (manifested by an increase in production of the short-range humoral stimulators of proliferation and differentiation of the erythroid progenitors) and activation of the erythropoietin system in the blood serum [46, 79, 115]. It should be also noted that the key roles in enhancement of blood EPA during inflammation are given to the substances released by the activated leukocytes in the inflammatory focus [125, 381]. When considering

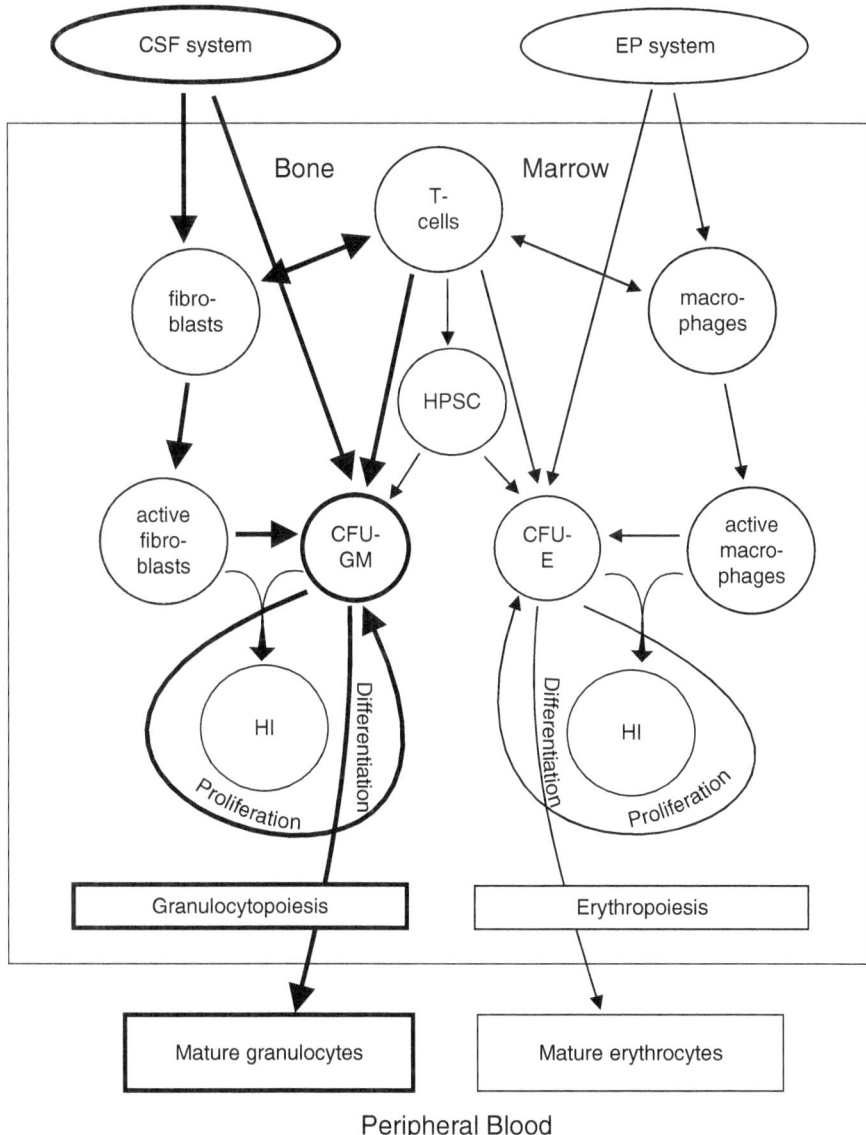

Fig. 2.2 Control of hematopoiesis during infectious inflammation. The fine continuous lines correspond to negligible effect on the indicated structures, while the heavy lines represent activation

the mechanisms of hemopoietic activation during inflammation, one should bear in mind that under these conditions as well as under the action of other stimulants, the bone marrow is invaded by migrating T-lymphocytes that stimulate the processes of proliferation and differentiation of the myeloid precursors CFU-GM and CFU-E either individually (via the release of their own lymphokines) or in cooperation with other HIM elements (specifically, with monocyte-macrophages) (Fig. 2.2).

It is corroborated by the fact that removal of Thy-1,2$^+$-cells from the bone marrow is accompanied by significant down-regulation of CFU-GM and CFU-E production, abrogation of up-regulation of CSA production by the adherent myelocaryocytes, and inhibition of CSA and EPA production by the non-adherent HIM elements.

In contrast, acute blood loss activates erythropoiesis, which becomes predominant among other changes of the medullar hemopoiesis. In rats, the blood loss of 1 % body weight elevated the total count of myelocaryocytes predominantly due to an increase in the total number of erythroid cells. The early terms of examination are characterized with stimulation of formation of the erythroid colonies that cannot be revealed during cloning the bone marrow of intact animals (without addition of erythropoietin into the culture medium). Moreover, the blood loss increases the score of erythroblastic islets in the bone marrow similar to what takes place during immobilization stress, but in the case of blood loss, this effect is more pronounced and long-lasting attesting to HIM activation (Fig. 2.3).

The development of hyperplasia of erythroid hemopoietic lineage in rats subjected to the blood loss is accompanied with corresponding increase in the counts of reticulocytes and erythrocytes in the peripheral blood. The study of erythropoietic properties of the blood serum drawn from experimental animals concluded that the degree of productive performance of erythron after blood loss and other perturbing stimuli is proportional to content of erythropoietin in the peripheral blood. These facts indicate existence of identical humoral mechanisms, which control proliferation and differentiation of the erythroid progenitor cells. How, during the blood loss the above changes in the level of erythropoietic activity of the blood are related predominantly to the developing circulatory and hemic hypoxia [42, 78, 249, 382]. It should be stressed that under the given experimental conditions, activation of erythropoiesis is accompanied by rather moderately expressed signs of the changes in the control over other myeloid lineages (elevation of serum CSA as well as up-regulation of proliferation and differentiation of the medullar granulocyte-macrophage progenitors), which stimulate the processes of granulomonocytopoiesis.

Thus, despite the fact that alterations in the blood system provoked by naturally diverse pathogenic factors and the mechanisms underlying these changes are virtually of the same type, the specific reaction of the blood system is determined by the nature of the acting stimulus.

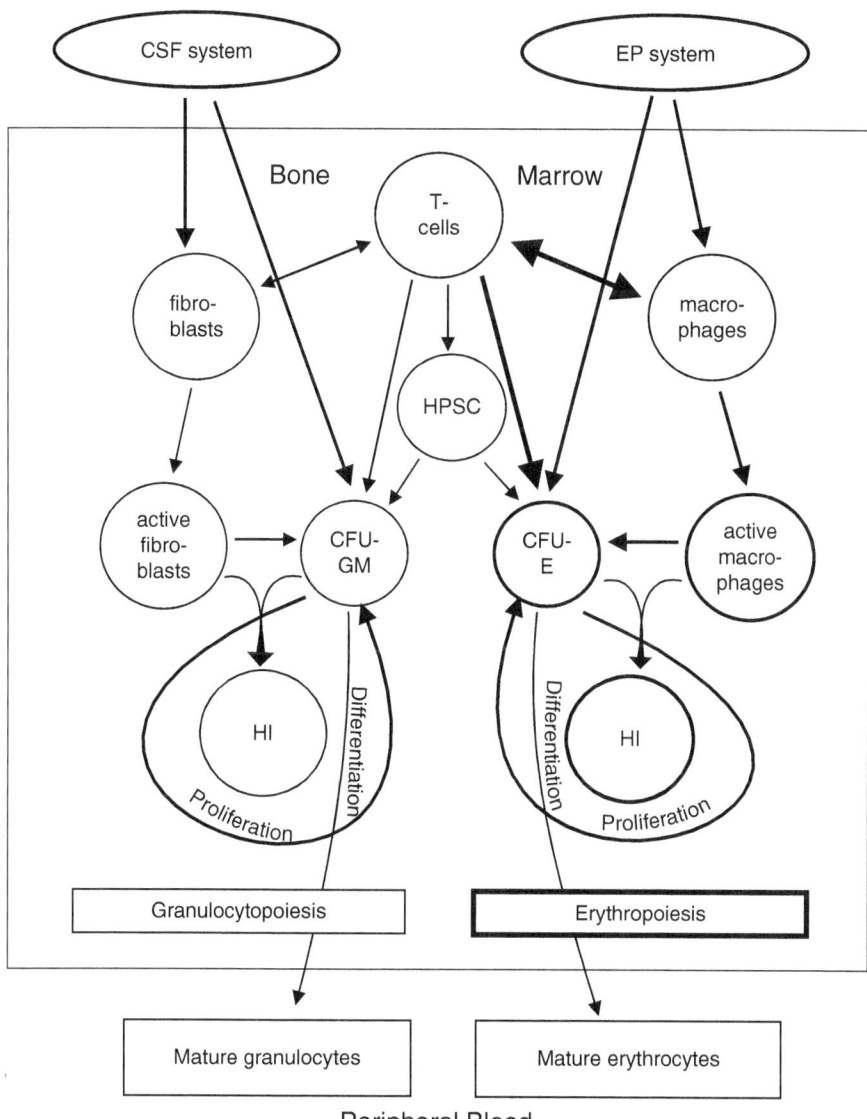

Fig. 2.3 Control of hematopoiesis during acute blood loss. Absence of any significant changes is marked with fine continuous lines, while the heavy lines represent activation

Chapter 3
Disturbances in Hemopoietic Control During Neurotic Disorders

At present, the experimental models of neurotic disorders have been developed, which are sufficiently good to reproduce clinical presentation of some neurosis forms, thereby opening the way to examine the pharmacological effects of antineurotic drugs. One of the popular models of a neurotic stimulation is the conflict situation based on 'collision' of the defensive and food-procuring reflexes, which in many respects is comparable to situation of uncertainty and to the state of insurmountable or difficult obstacle in humans [116, 161]. Another example of such models is deprivation of the paradoxical sleep, which exerts specific (first of all, in relation to memory and cognitive functions) asthenizing effect on CNS, because the paradoxical phase of sleep plays the key role in information processing [11, 66, 117, 282]. The sleep requirements result from necessity to block the sensory input in order to process and integrate the daily portion of information obtained by the brain. This model simulates many features of CNS asthenization provoked in patients by diverse pathologies including the neurotic disorders resulting from sleep deprivation. Moreover, deprivation of the paradoxical sleep shapes the peculiar state of CNS, which inhibits the active search behavior in wakeful animals. Under sleep deprivation model, the animal cannot compensate this behavioral abnormality by normal paradoxical sleep. The long-term deficiency in search activity culminates in the death of animals [117].

Our study of the reactions of blood system and the mechanisms of their development during experimental neuroses showed that the conflict situation and deprivation of paradoxical sleep provoke pronounced and unequal shifts in the indices describing the bone marrow and peripheral blood [47, 86, 87, 144, 160–162].

One of the basic features of hematopoiesis during neurotic influences is its phasic character. It is noteworthy that at the early terms of observation (days 1–3 after the onset of stimulation), the changes in the blood system are unspecific and relate to triggering the redistributive mechanisms [86, 87, 161]. The observed integral response comprising activation of granulocytopoiesis, inhibition of the lymphoid lineage, neutrophilic leukocytosis, and reticulocytosis in the peripheral blood is in many respects comparable to the development of 'emergency defense' at the early

© Springer International Publishing Switzerland 2014
A.M. Dygai, V.V. Zhdanov, *Theory of Hematopoiesis Control*,
SpringerBriefs in Cell Biology 5, DOI 10.1007/978-3-319-08584-5_3

period of the stress reaction [59, 60, 78]. The second observation period (days 4–7 after neurotic stimulation) was characterized with the specific changes in some lineages. In particular, the conflict situation induced hyperplasia of bone marrow hemopoiesis and neutrophilic leukocytosis as well as lymphocytosis and reticulocytosis in the peripheral blood [86, 87, 161]. Deprivation of the paradoxical sleep stimulated the development of granulocyte lineage to a far lesser extent than that observed during conflict situation, and it was accompanied with chronic depression of erythron and lymphopoiesis.

Our studies showed that important role in plastic rearrangement of medullar hemopoiesis under the neurotic influences is given to the pool of hemopoietic progenitor cells. The conflict situation up-regulates proliferative activity and intensity of differentiation of erythroid and granulomonocyte precursor cells [47, 85, 160]. In contrast, deprivation of the paradoxical sleep inhibits division and maturation of the erythroid cells, which is accompanied by desynchronization of the processes in the pool of granulomonocyte precursor cells.

Thus, under the considered neurotic influences and during exposure of an organism to diverse stress factors (infectious inflammation, immobilization, acute blood loss, hemolytic anemia, *etc*.), the changes in intensity of proliferation and differentiation of the committed hemopoietic progenitor cells play important role in selection of direction and the depth of disturbances in the blood system [40]. In its turn, proliferation and differentiation of the stem cells are controlled by sophisticated multilayer regulation system, which includes the distant (based on the neurotransmitters) and local mechanisms.

We revealed the key role of the core subdivisions of CNS in the formation of the hematological alterations during experimental neurotic stimulation. Under these conditions, transmission of the instructive information from CNS to hematopoietic cells is effected both directly via adrenergic structures on the hemopoietic precursors and indirectly via α- and β-adrenergic receptors on HIM cellular elements. At the same time, the performance of hematopoietic progenitors in many respects depends on the medullar T-lymphocytes that express Thy-1,2 antigen on its surface.

The experiments showed that depletion of the catecholamine depot with reserpine or pharmacological blockade of α- and β-adrenergic structures with dihydroergotamine and propranolol prevented the development of hyperplasia of the medullar hemopoiesis during the conflict situation, which was accompanied by the corresponding changes in the state of peripheral blood. In its turn, reserpine augmented inhibition of medullar erythropoiesis provoked by deprivation of the paradoxical sleep, while dihydroergotamine and propranolol restored activity of the erythroid hemopoietic lineage. Stimulation of α- and β-adrenergic receptors by phenylephrine and orciprenaline sulfate activated the inhibited erythropoiesis up to the state of hyperplasia, enhanced granulocytopoiesis, and additionally stimulated the hematopoietic processes during the conflict situation [48, 171].

Pharmacological blockade of vegetative ganglia with pentamine aggravated depression of erythropoiesis provoked by deprivation of the paradoxical sleep and inhibited it during the conflict situation. It is interesting that pentamine up-regulated hyperplasia of granulocytopoiesis during deprivation of the paradoxical sleep but down-regulated it under the conflict situation [170].

Pharmacological blockade of dopamine and serotonin postsynaptic receptors with respectively, haloperidol and cyproheptadine as well as inhibition of the M-cholinergic structures with scopolamine down-regulated hyperplasia of medullar erythro- and granulocytopoiesis in animals subjected to the conflict situation. In contrast, during deprivation of the paradoxical sleep the pharmacological blockade of these structures abrogated depression of medullar erythropoiesis [57].

Thus, under the conflict situation the 'positive' effects of adrenergic, M-cholinergic, and serotoninergic systems stimulate functional activity of HIM elements, proliferation and differentiation of the hemopoietic progenitors. The direct and indirect (mediated by interaction with adherent HIM elements such as macrophages and the stromal mechanocytes) potencies of the regulator T-cells to stimulate the growth of hemopoietic precursors have been demonstrated (Fig. 3.1) [168, 169].

Simultaneously, cooperation of Thy-1,2$^+$-cells with macrophages and the stromal mechanocytes induces a cascade of the changes in the system of local regulation of hematopoiesis manifested by up-regulation of HI formation and production of hemopoietins by the HIM cellular elements, which in its turn stimulates division and maturation of the erythroid and granulomonocyte precursor cells and up-regulates the hemopoietic hyperplasia [47, 160].

Deprivation of the paradoxical sleep depletes the central monoaminergic regulator mechanisms, which similar to the inhibitory effect of M-cholinergic systems limit the interaction of Thy-1,2$^+$-cells with the elements of adherent fraction in the bone marrow and inhibit binding of CFU-E and CFU-GM with the stromal cells (Fig. 3.2).

The final results of disturbances of the cell-cell interactions are manifested by inhibition of the formation of auxiliary foci of erythroid hemopoiesis, depression of secretion of the humoral stimulators of hematopoiesis by adherent HIM fraction, desynchronization of proliferation and differentiation of the granulocyte-macrophage precursor cells, and down-regulation of mitotic activity and maturation of the erythroid cells. This cascade of alterations culminates in the development of 'abortive' hyperplasia of granulocytopoiesis and long-term depression of erythropoiesis. In these processes, the serotoninergic system is mostly responsible for the changes in erythropoiesis, while the dopaminergic system is mainly involved in alterations of granulocytopoiesis [47, 160].

Therefore, in conflict situation the hematopoietic microenvironment works according to 'stress type'. The mechanisms of inhibitory effect of deprivation of the paradoxical sleep on hemopoiesis are related to the disturbances in cell-cell interactions between the individual cell elements in HIM (T-cells, macrophages, stromal mechanocytes) and the hemopoietic precursor cells.

Our studies revealed the important features of medullar hemopoiesis in the intact mice with active and passive behavior as well as the specific interactions between HIM and the monoaminergic systems in the control of functional activity of the hemopoietic progenitor cells during experimental neuroses [49, 144, 169].

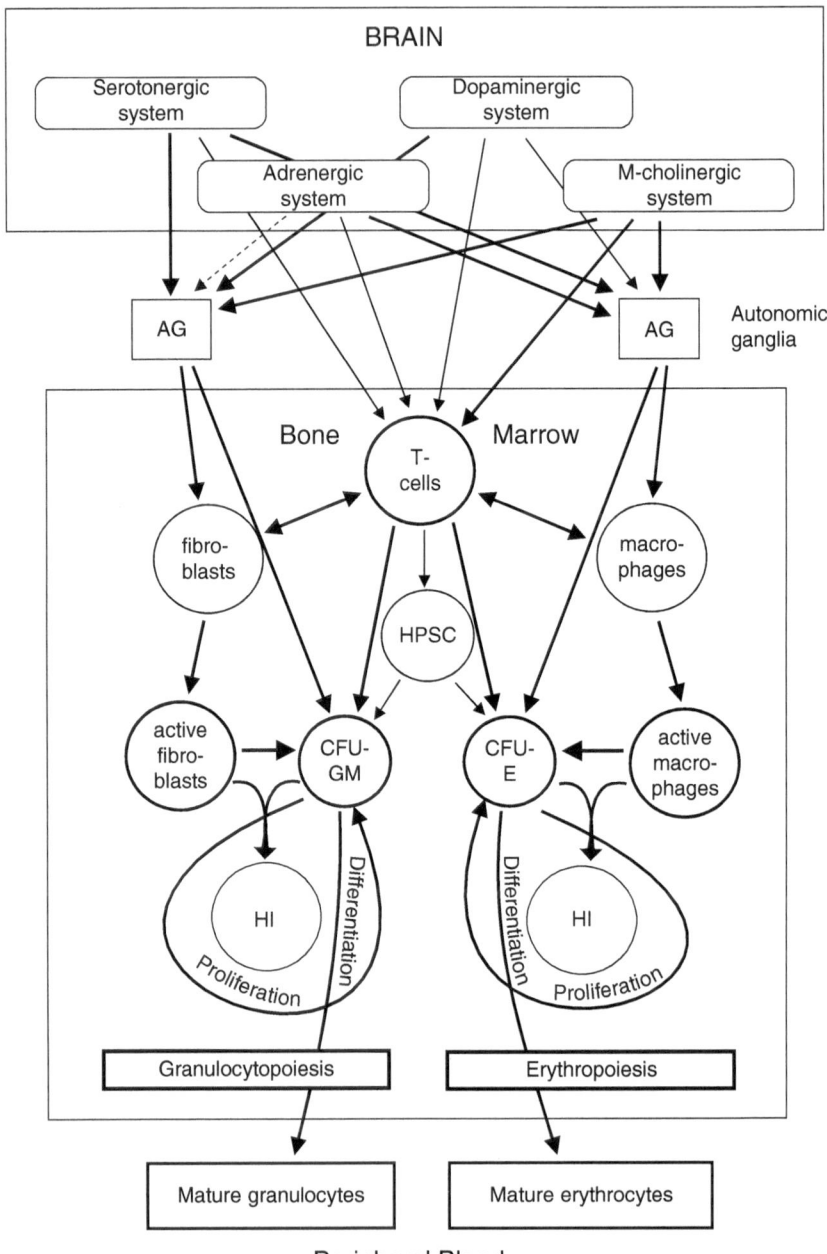

Fig. 3.1 Control of hematopoiesis in the conflict situation. Absence of any significant changes is marked with fine continuous lines, while the *dash* and *thick solid lines* indicate inhibition and activation, correspondingly

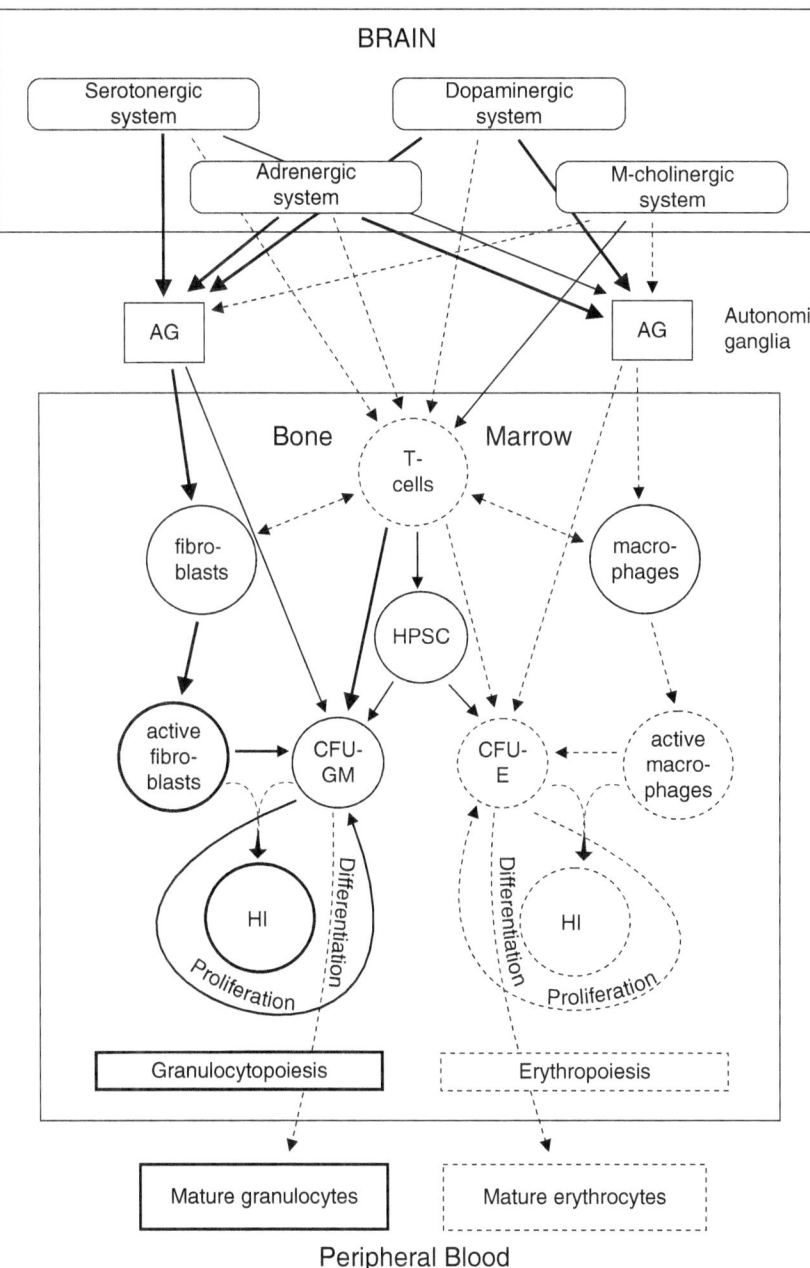

Fig. 3.2 Control of hematopoiesis during deprivation of the paradoxical sleep. Absence of any significant changes is marked with fine continuous lines, while the *dash* and *thick solid lines* indicate inhibition and activation, correspondingly

The peculiarities of hemopoiesis in intact active and passive mice are determined by the intergroup differences in the structure-functional organization of the bone marrow and intensity of proliferation and differentiation of the granulocyte-macrophage precursor cells mediated via α-adrenergic structures. In active mice subjected to the conflict situation, up-regulation of HI formation, enhancement of the production of humoral hemopoietic regulators by HIM elements, and increase in the count of blood serum hemopoietins induce synchronous elevation in the rates of division and maturation of the progenitor cells (mediated via the α-adrenergic structures), which leads to the development of pronounced hyperplasia of the medullar hemopoiesis. Simultaneously, the mutual influence augments between the compartments of the erythroid and granulocyte hemopoiesis and between the HIM elements and the precursor cells. Deprivation of the paradoxical sleep in active mice inhibits the formation of all types of cell associations resulting in deficiency of the hemopoietic growth factors in the blood serum where CSA is greater affected than EPA. In its turn, this deficiency inhibits and desynchronizes proliferation and differentiation of the hematopoietic precursor cells culminating in the development of depression of the medullar hemopoiesis.

The corner stones in the development of hematopoietic hypoplasia in passive mice during the conflict situation are degraded bone marrow ability to form any kind of the cell associations, disturbance in secretion of the hemopoietic growth factors by the adherent cells of the hemopoietic microenvironment, and finally, inhibition and desynchronization (via the α-adrenergic structures) of division and maturation of the erythropoietic precursor cells. In passive mice subjected to deprivation of the paradoxical sleep, two opposite processes are going on: (1) up-regulation of the formation of auxiliary foci of granulocytic hemopoiesis and enhancement of CSA secretion by the HIM cellular elements and (2) down-regulation of the formation of erythroid cell associations, moderation of EPA secretion by the elements of hemopoietic microenvironment, as well as abatement of functional activity of the erythroid precursor cells.

The correlation analysis revealed strong dependence of functional activity of the erythropoietic precursor cells on the adrenergic structures in active mice stimulated by the conflict situation and in passive mice deprived of the paradoxical sleep. In other groups, desynchronization of division and maturation of the erythroid colony- and cluster-forming units was less related to the adrenergic stimulation, while the disturbances in the division and maturation of granulocyte-macrophage precursor cells were mostly related to α-adrenergic regulation.

Overall, the considered data attest to existence of two potential therapeutic avenues to minimize the pathogenic consequences of the neurotic influences. One way is to enhance neurotic tolerance of the patients, while the second approach is to moderate the neurotic alterations in CNS and in the effector organs such as the blood system.

Chapter 4
Alterations in the Blood System During Myelosuppression Induced by Cytostatic and Radiation Treatment

The hematopoietic tissue belongs to the structures extremely sensitive to the action of antiblastomic drugs and ionizing radiation, which is explained mostly by a high proliferative activity of its constituent elements, so this system is the gold standard model to examine the regularities in the development of biological effects and the modes of action of the myeloinhibitory agents [9, 15, 21, 22, 143, 153, 207, 262, 267, 309]. However, the search for most rational and efficient ways to correct the hypoplastic manifestations should be based on more detailed knowledge about the mechanisms of suppression and recovery of hematopoiesis in patients subjected to radiation and cytostatic therapy.

Alterations in the blood system observed during the development of cytostatic and radiation diseases were examined in a great number of experimental works. Modern science accumulated numerous data on the state of the major subdivisions of hematopoietic tissue in experimental animals subjected to radiation and administered with different doses of antitumor drugs [6, 24, 58, 127, 208, 212, 224, 242, 263, 306]. However, interpretation of these data in respect to deciphering the mechanisms of recovery of the suppressed hemopoiesis does not encompass all the important features of regenerative processes in the hematopoietic tissue. Specifically, replenishment of the morphologically identified cells in the bone marrow can be effected either by reproduction of the hematopoietic elements that survived after the cytostatic therapy or by employing the less mature progenitor cells [112, 118, 205, 278]. It should be stressed that such important avenue of hemopoietic reparation as accelerated differentiation of the hemopoietic precursor cells under the conditions of suppressed cell proliferation received little attention.

Analysis of the present data revealed significant differences in the depth and duration of hemopoietic depression after the use of various cytostatic drugs and radiation therapy in the doses that are equivalent in the matter of general biological effect [12, 17, 58, 207, 212, 263, 267, 306]. Usually, these paradoxical differences are explained by unequal damage to the hematopoietic cells exerted by the myeloinhibitory agents with diverse modes of action. The toxic effect towards the hematopoietic elements is surely the most important feature, which

© Springer International Publishing Switzerland 2014
A.M. Dygai, V.V. Zhdanov, *Theory of Hematopoiesis Control*,
SpringerBriefs in Cell Biology 5, DOI 10.1007/978-3-319-08584-5_4

determines the character of myelosuppressive effect in any particular case. However, little attention was focused to the changes in the functional state of the regulatory apparatus of the hematopoietic tissue provoked by the antiblastomic drugs, which most surely contribute to the specific manifestations of the cytostatic and radiation diseases.

The most important role in the control of hematopoiesis in the norm and diverse extreme influences is played by HIM composed of various types of the cell elements and extracellular matrix. HIM exerts the local control over proliferation and differentiation of the hemopoietic cells by releasing the humoral factors and by transmitting the signals during the direct cell-cell interactions [90, 95, 96, 123, 198, 229, 266, 313, 320, 359, 370, 371]. At the same time, the cells of hemopoietic microenvironment are rather sensitive to the cytostatic drugs and ionizing radiation [52, 93, 137, 200, 206, 211, 232, 285, 342, 364, 383].

In addition, the plasmatic membrane of hematopoietic progenitor cells at different maturation levels as well as the morphologically identified hemopoietic and stromal cells can expose the receptors to different transmitters (such as acetylcholine, catecholamines, serotonin, substance P, opioids, *etc.*). The studies revealed direct (receptive) and indirect (mediated via HIM cell elements) regulatory effects of neurotransmitters on proliferation and differentiation of the committed precursors of hemopoiesis [96, 215, 323, 352, 374]. Most probably, these data indicate existence of monoaminergic control over the processes of damage and regeneration of the hematopoietic tissue during myeloinhibitory influences.

Overall, the study of the roles played by HIM with its elements and by central and peripheral monoamines in sustaining the hemopoietic regenerative processes can help to develop the pathogenically reasonable ways to correct the disturbances in the blood system provoked by the antiblastomic therapy.

Under extreme influences leading to hypoplasia of the hematopoietic tissue (radiation, the use of cytostatic drugs in the doses that are equivalent by the general biological effect), hemopoietic recovery develops in various ways. Along with the direct suppressive effects of the toxic agents on hematopoietic cells, the recovery dynamics of hematopoiesis is mostly determined by the character of hematopoietic disorders. First of all, one should bear in mind the changes in functional activity of individual HIM elements [2, 40, 53, 179, 250]. For example, a single total irradiation of mice at a dose of 2.0 Gy provoked the development of the bone marrow variant of acute radiation sickness. The total cellularity of the bone marrow decreased to the end of day 1 after irradiation due to dramatic drop in the content of erythroid elements, immature neutrophils, and the lymphoid cells (on the average, by 70 % initial level). In 2 days, the bone marrow displayed the first signs of hemopoietic regeneration manifested by appearance of the immature forms of myeloid cells such as myeloblasts and promyelocytes. To the end of experiment day 4, the complete recovery of the total number of myelocaryocytes and cellularity of all hematopoietic lineages took place. The peripheral blood indices attained the initial values on experiment day 7 [2, 69].

A rather gradual and not especially intensive reparation of granulocytic and erythroid medullar lineages after exposure to ionizing radiation is explained by the

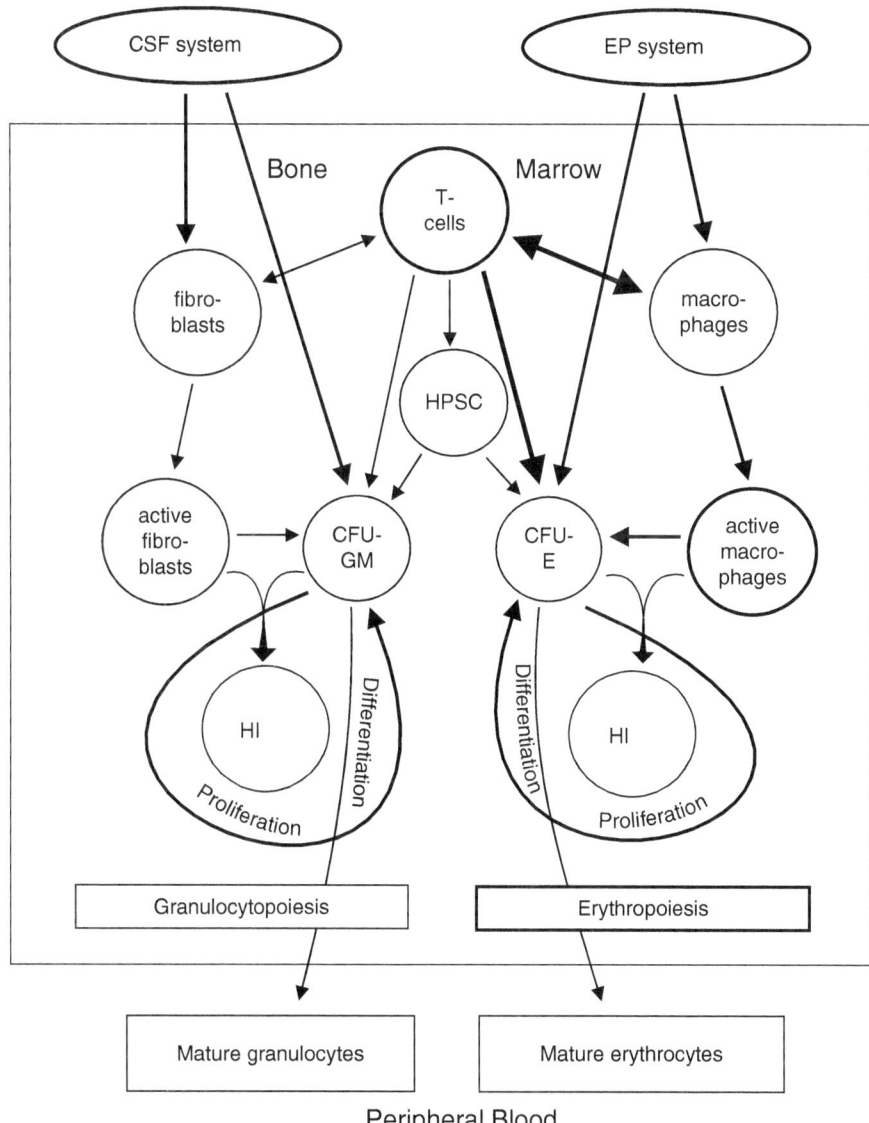

Fig. 4.1 Control of hematopoiesis during myelosuppression caused by total irradiation. Absence of any significant changes is marked with fine continuous lines, while the *dash* and *thick solid lines* indicate inhibition and activation, correspondingly

fact that the total irradiation produces no significant changes in the functional activity of HIM elements (Fig. 4.1).

Elevation of serum CSA and EPA accelerates proliferation of the corresponding precursors. The absence of any drastic changes in maturation of hemopoietic elements results from a rather stable structure-functional state of the hematopoietic tissue. Stimulation of direct and indirect (mediated via macrophage system) mechanisms of the erythropoietic control exerted by T-cells results in acceleration of erythron recovery [2].

When administered at MTD, the most cytostatic drugs produce pronounced myeloinhibitory effect manifested by decreased cellularity of bone marrow and some hematopoietic lineages. In mice, the most pronounced and long-lasting depletion of the hematopoietic tissue was observed after injection of **5-fluorouracil**. In our studies, the maximum of depression was observed on experiment day 5 when the total count of myelocaryocytes was merely 6.3 % initial level. Slow recovery of hematopoiesis finished only to experiment day 14. Chronic inhibition of granulocytic and erythroid medullar lineages by 5-fluorouracil was accompanied by elevation of the content of the committed precursors in hematopoietic tissue resulting from the disturbances in the processes of their maturation [37, 53, 384] (Fig. 4.2).

This phenomenon resulted from stimulation of proliferation of the hemopoietic precursor cells against the background of unrestored (due to pronounced dissociation of the progenitors and the stromal elements of the microenvironment) structure-functional organization of the bone marrow. Under these conditions, up-regulation of proliferative activity of the clonogenic cells results from an increase in secretion of the hemopoietic growth factors by T-cells during the late terms of experiment due to their accumulation in the hematopoietic region and interaction with the adherent elements.

Under these conditions, the adrenergic system plays a positive role in the processes of hemopoietic tissue regeneration due to activation of HI formation, up-regulation of EPA production by HIM non-adherent cells, and elevation of serum CSA. On the one hand, the dopaminergic system increases the rate of erythron regeneration by raising the level of serum EPA and by increasing the erythropoietin-dependent activation of CFU-E proliferation, and on the other hand, it delays the recovery of granulocytic hemopoietic lineage due to down-regulation of CSA production by the adherent cells in the hemopoietic microenvironment. In its turn, the serotoninergic system augments the development of erythropoiesis depression due to down-regulation of EPA secretion by the adherent cells in HIM, although it increases the recovery rate of the granulocytic hemopoietic lineage by up-regulating formation of the granulocyte and mixt HI and by stimulating division and maturation of the granulomonocytic precursors mediated via the system of the colony-stimulating factors [84, 128, 129, 163, 165].

The changes in the content of the medullar hemopoietic cells in animals treated with anthracycline antibiotic **adriamycin** were biphasic in character. On postinjection days 2–4, the count of medullar nucleated cells decreased, which was followed by a transient rise to initial level and subsequent drop on days 9–11. The study of the mechanisms of hematopoietic recovery showed that activation of differentiation of the committed progenitors triggered by adriamycin and the consequential rapid regeneration of the hemopoietic tissue (Fig. 4.3) resulted from the leading recovery of medullar HI and especially from their intensive formation by the mature macrophages.

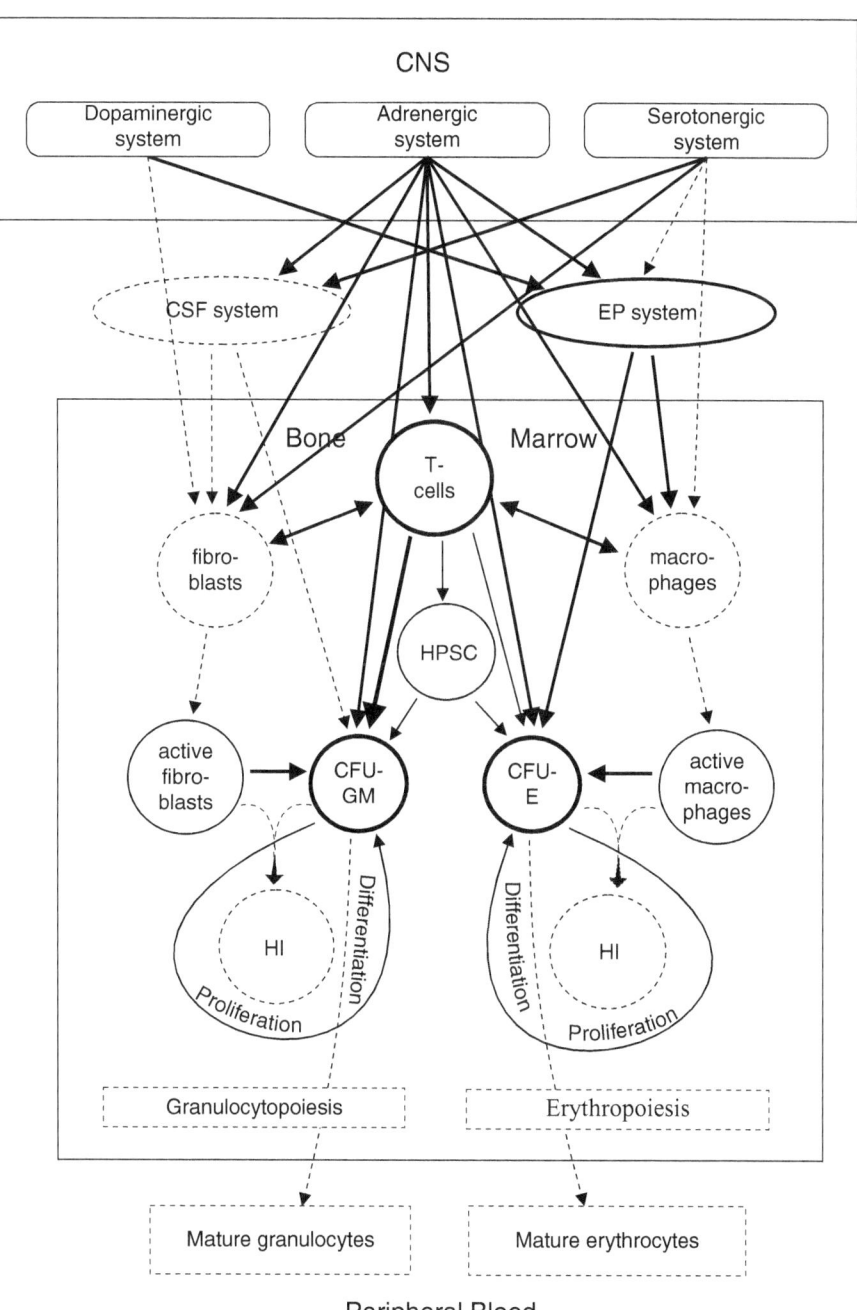

Fig. 4.2 Control of hematopoiesis during myelosuppression caused by injection of fluoropyrimidine antimetabolite 5-fluorouracil. Absence of any significant changes is marked with fine continuous lines, while the *dash* and *thick solid lines* indicate inhibition and activation, correspondingly

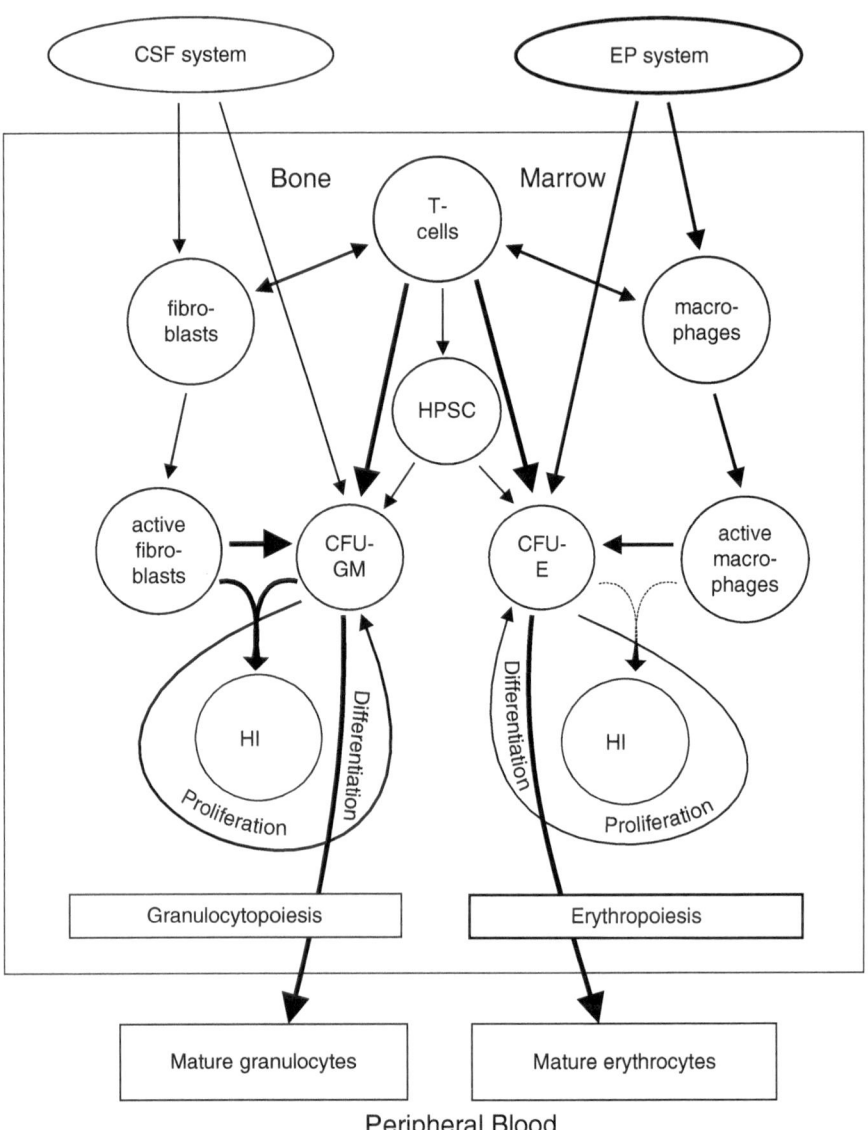

Fig. 4.3 Control of hematopoiesis during myelosuppression caused by injection of anthracycline antibiotic adriamycin. Absence of any significant changes is marked with fine continuous lines, while the *dash* and *thick solid lines* indicate inhibition and activation, correspondingly

In addition, an important role is played by stimulation of the coupling between the stromal mechanocytes and hemopoietic precursor cells [37]. At this, the high level of proliferative activity of hemopoietic precursors results from up-regulation of production of the hemopoiesis-stimulating activities by microenvironmental elements at the early terms of examination promoted by vigorous recovery of their population.

Cyclophosphane also induced rapid reparation of the structure-functional organization of the bone marrow and early up-regulation of secretory activity of the adherent myelocaryocytes in cooperation with T-cells, which provided accelerated transition of the granulocyte-macrophage precursor cells to differentiation phase [37]. As a result, the total score of medullar cell rapidly restored mostly due to active regeneration of the granulocytic hemopoietic lineage. The content of immature forms of the neutrophilic granulocytes assessed on day 2 after injection of the alkylating agent was as low as 3.5 % initial level, but on day 5, the number of these cells increased almost 3-fold in comparison with initial level, and their count remained elevated to the end of experiment. In a natural way, the content of mature medullar neutrophils attained maximum to day 8, and it normalized during subsequent 4 days. At the same time, the long-term decrease in the content of erythrocaryocyte is probably explained by pronounced damaging effect of the alkylating agent exerted directly to the committed precursors of the erythroid hemopoietic lineage [37, 112].

The dopaminergic system predominantly augments the disturbances in the structure-functional organization of the erythroid compartment of hemopoiesis caused by the alkylating agent, which results in additional delay in regeneration of erythropoiesis and in more pronounced reticulocytopenia in the peripheral blood [128, 165]. These processes are accompanied by stimulation of G-CSF- and dopamine-dependent control mechanisms over proliferation of granulomonocytic progenitors impeding the development of neutrophilic leukopenia [84, 163].

The inhibitory effect of adrenergic system on granulocytic and erythroid hemopoietic lineages under the action of cyclophosphane (Fig. 4.4) is mediated via inhibition of functional activity of the HIM adherent cells (i.e., by down-regulating HI formation and EPA production) as well as via decrease in the division rate of granulomonocytic progenitors related to G-CSF and peripheral adrenergic mechanisms.

Additional down-regulating effect of the serotoninergic system on the erythron is related to inhibition of formation of the erythroid HI, moderation of functional activity of the erythroid progenitors (mediated by the erythropoietin system), and decrease in the level of EPA produced by auxiliary bone marrow cells [129, 165, 166].

Etoposide (a derivative of podophyllotoxin) decreased the total score of myelocaryocytes on postinjection days 1–7, but on day 8, this score elevated to 121.5 % initial value (Fig. 4.5). In the following, this parameter decreased again attaining the initial value to postinjection day 12. Examination of myelogram showed that the drop in the total bone marrow cellularity resulted from a decrease in the content of mature forms of neutrophilic granulocytes, nucleated erythroid cells, lymphoid elements, and monocyte-macrophages.

Accumulation of the progenitors of erythro- and granulomonocytopoiesis in the bone marrow due to differentiation of less mature cells developed in parallel with intensive recovery of the corresponding hemopoietic lineages [89, 179, 110]. At this, elevation in cellularity of the hematopoietic tissue was mostly provided by activation of maturation of the committed precursors. This process was caused by

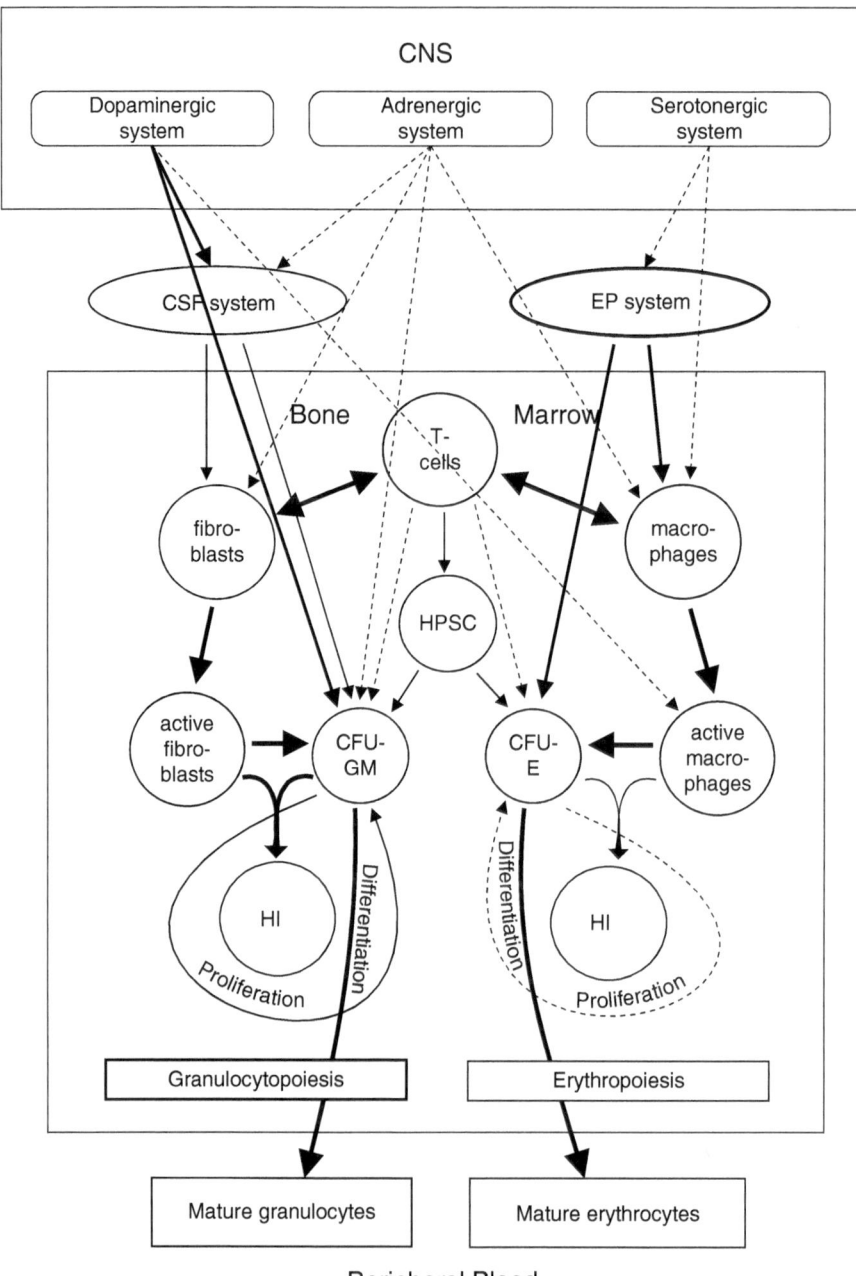

Fig. 4.4 Control of hematopoiesis during myelosuppression caused by alkylating agent cyclophosphane. Absence of any significant changes is marked with fine continuous lines, while the *dash* and *thick solid lines* indicate inhibition and activation, correspondingly

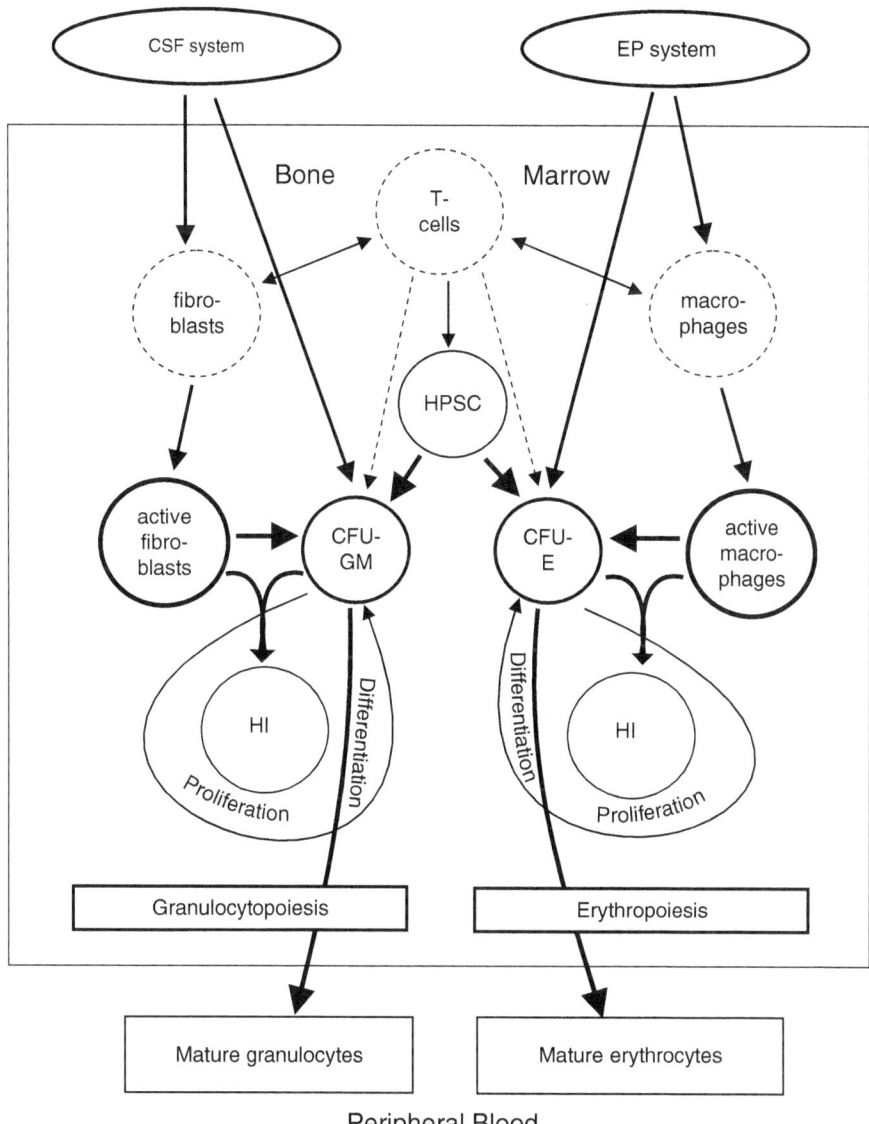

Fig. 4.5 Control of hematopoiesis during myelosuppression caused by etoposide, a derivative of podophyllotoxin. Absence of any significant changes is marked with fine continuous lines, while the *dash* and *thick solid lines* indicate inhibition and activation, correspondingly

augmented adhesive potency of the elements in the hematopoietic microenvironment towards the colony-forming cells accompanied by elevated score of the growth factors in the blood serum and by active production of the colony-stimulating factors by the adherent cells in the bone marrow [179].

Carboplatin provoked anemia and thrombocytopenia even at the early terms after injection. Decrease in the content of erythrocytes and hemoglobin in the peripheral blood resulted from a pronounced inhibition of medullar hemopoiesis on postinjection days 5–12 [194]. At this, leucopoiesis was damaged to a small degree, the alterations being observed only at the later terms of examination. Under the absence of adequate reaction of the distant humoral system (erythropoietin) to cytostatic damage produced by this nephrotoxic agent, there was an up-regulation in secretion of the erythropoiesis-stimulating humoral factors by the adherent cells in HIM. Such activation of the local mechanisms resulted in accumulation of erythroid progenitors in the bone marrow, but it could not ensure efficient recovery of the erythron (Fig. 4.6).

Thus, the character of hematopoietic recovery under the action of various myelo-inhibitory agents significantly depends on peculiarities of the disturbances in the hemopoietic control provoked by applied agent. It is explained by the fact that intensity of growth and maturation of the hematopoietic cells during regeneration are determined by the damage of specific elements in HIM. For example, the use of 5-fluorouracil is characterized with disturbance of functional activity of the cells in the system of mononuclear phagocytes with relative functional integrity of the T-lymphocyte system [40, 53, 385]. In contrast, cyclophosphane is notorious for pronounced toxicity against T-cells [37, 57, 386]. In both cases, dysregulation of hematopoiesis results from uncoupling of the cooperative interaction between T-lymphocytes and macrophages in regulation of the cell cycle in the pool of pro-genitor cells, which is accompanied by prevalence of the corresponding processes according to proliferation and differentiation of these cells. Under the conditions of perturbed cell-cell cooperative interactions between various HIM elements, the activity of hematopoietic tissue is shaped by the spectrum of humoral agents (cytokines and GAG) secreted by these elements. In other words, in similar situa-tions T-lymphocytes can control the proliferative processes (specifically, via IL-3 production), while the adherent cell can regulate differentiation of the cells (for example, via production of IL-1 and the lineage-restricted hemopoietins).

Disturbances in the hematopoietic mechanisms are also caused by radiation, although they are expressed to a far smaller degree than those produced by 5-fluorouracil and cyclophosphane [2, 387]. Correspondingly, the radiation-induced changes in the control of hematopoiesis do not significantly impede regeneration of the hematopoietic tissue.

Under the action of adriamycin or etoposide, the overall changes in hemopoietic microenvironment induced by cytostatic drugs promote the hemopoietic recovery pro-cesses. Thus, in these particular cases, these changes play the positive adaptive role.

In hypoplastic states resulting from the use of cytostatic drugs, the adrenergic, dopaminergic, and serotoninergic pathways control (1) proliferation and differentia-tion of the committed hemopoietic progenitors in HIM, (2) functional activity of HIM cell elements, (3) the system of colony-stimulating factors, and (4) the erythropoietin system. At this, the serotoninergic system is mostly responsible for alterations in erythroid hemopoietic lineage, while the adrenergic and dopaminergic systems pre-dominantly affect the granulocytic hemopoietic lineage [165, 167, 172].

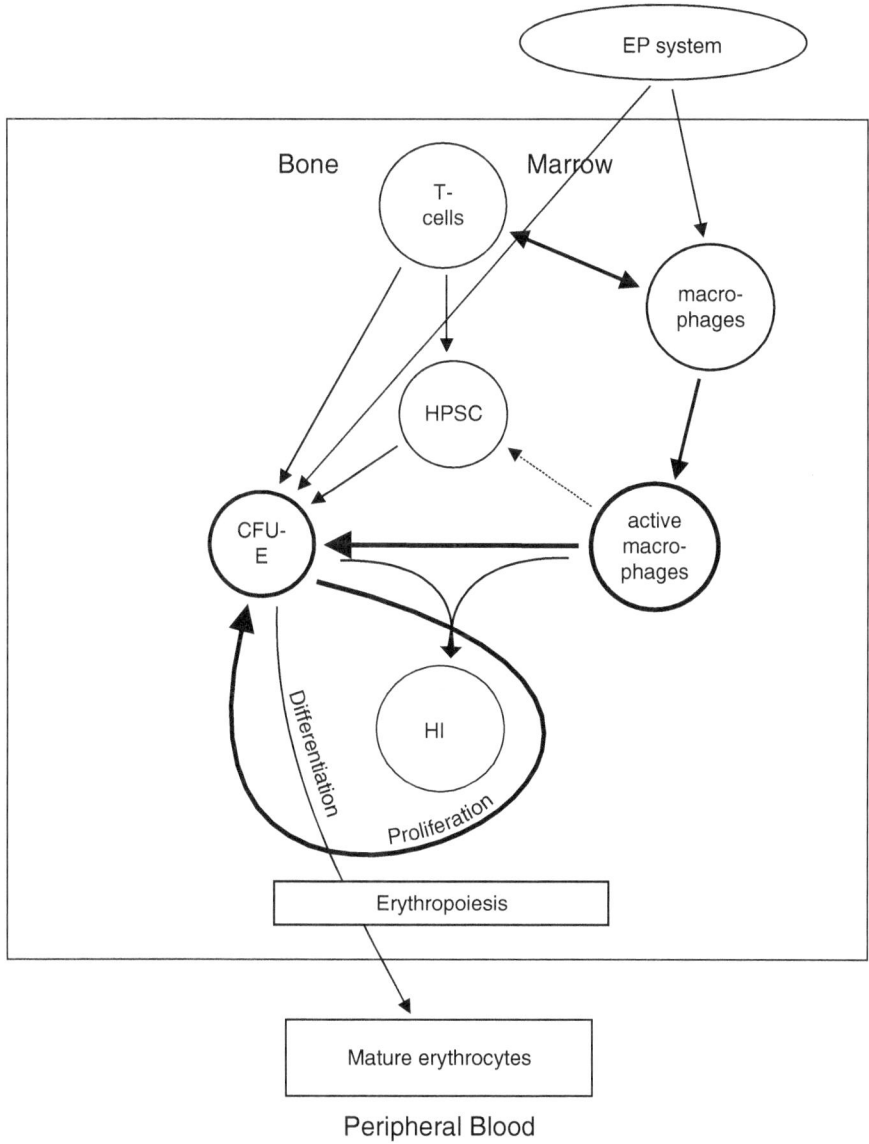

Fig. 4.6 Control of erythropoiesis during myelosuppression caused by carboplatin. Absence of any significant changes is marked with fine continuous lines, while the *dash* and *thick solid lines* indicate inhibition and activation, correspondingly

Examination of these control mechanisms showed that the ligands of monoaminergic nature (predominantly, α- and β-adrenomimetics) accelerate differentiation of the pluripotent hemopoietic cells into progenitors of granulomonocytopoiesis (induced by G-CSF *in vitro*) and increase the rate of division of the newly formed

CFU-GM. At the same time, the monoaminergic transmitters (typically, serotonin) enhance the feeder activity of the fibroblastic elements for CFU-G [172].

Reserpine-induced potentiation of granulocytopoiesis-stimulating activity of G-CSF under the action of cyclophosphane is explained by elevation of the content of the pluripotent hemopoietic cells, by increased rate of their differentiation towards the progenitors of granulomonocytopoiesis, and by the stimulating effect of the stromal elements and Thy-1.2$^+$-cells on the hemopoietic progenitors (predominantly, on CFU-GEMM) [82, 83].

In view of progressive improvements of the methods employed in treatment of the malignant neoplasms and increase in the number of the long-living patients, one of the central problems in tumor chemotherapy can be the long-term side effects of the toxic action of cytostatic drugs on the normal (not affected by the tumor) and actively proliferating cell systems. While the disturbances in nervous, cardiovascular, and endocrine systems can be rather easily detected and diagnosticated, the changes in the blood system can be latent with the manifestations observed only during additional hematopoiesis-disturbing influences [58, 325].

For example, exposure of mice to immobilization stress in 1, 3, and 6 months after injection of **doxorubicin** and **vinblastine** in MTD induced pronounced changes in the parameters of hemopoietic control mechanisms. Injection of antitumor drugs enhanced responsiveness of the hematopoietic tissue in 1 month. In 6 months postinjection, the compensatory and adaptive reactions of the bone marrow to immobilization stress were little expressed or entirely absent. A single injection of cytostatic drugs in MTD depleted the pool of the committed progenitor cells at the late terms of this study. While in 1 month after injection of cytostatic drugs, the adequate reaction of the precursors to the additional hemopoiesis-perturbing influences was still observed, the reaction of the committed progenitors to immobilization stress was disturbed 5 months later. The long-term side effects of the damaging action of vinblastine and doxorubicin on hematopoiesis included diminished feeder activity of the adherent elements of the bone marrow. The characteristic abnormalities revealed in 1, 3, and 6 months after injection of vinblastine and doxorubicin were the changes in the content of medullar Thy-1,2$^+$-cells and disturbance of their migration into the bone marrow during additional hematopoiesis-perturbing influences.

The long-term side effects of toxic action of the antitumor drugs also include rearrangement of the short-range hemopoietic control mechanisms. In 1 month after injection of such drugs, an enhanced level of production of IL-3 activity is observed, while in 6 months, synthesis of IL-3 is pronouncedly down-regulated in contrast to up-regulated production of IL-1. The major reasons of hematopoietic disturbances observed at the later terms after injection of the antitumor preparations are the disturbances in functional activity of the stromal elements in the hemopoietic organs and consequential involvement of the interaction mechanisms between the hematopoietic cells and HIM cell elements into these pathologic changes.

The common unspecific features such as migration of T-lymphocytes into the bone marrow and activation of HIM and hemopoietic precursors which are characteristic of the stress reaction and hemopoiesis-suppressing extreme influences [2, 40, 44, 78, 86, 90], raise a problem of existence of certain universal neuro-endocrine mechanisms of physiological and reparative regeneration in the hematopoietic tissue.

Really, in addition to significant disorganization in the structure-functional integrity of the hematopoietic tissue, the disturbances in the hematopoietic control provoked by hemopoiesis-inhibitory influences (cytostatic drugs, ionizing radiation, *etc.*) include a pronounced neuroendocrine component related to activation of the stress-mediating systems of an organism [51, 53, 233]. However, in contrast to 'pure' stress reaction, these disturbances are characterized with elimination of cause-and-effect interrelations between the sympathoadrenal and blood systems. Moreover, the adrenergic transmitters aggravate uncoupling of the hematopoietic mechanisms, which is characteristic of the hematopoiesis-suppressive stimulants, because in contrast to stimulation of relatively resistant cells of the blood system, they inhibit reparation of the hemopoietic precursors and HIM elements damaged by the extreme influences. Finally, uncoupling of the hematopoietic mechanisms decreases the rate of regeneration of the hematopoietic tissue.

In particular, the catecholamines administered to the animals pre-treated with the high doses of 5-fluorouracil up-regulate proliferation and differentiation of CFU-E and CFU-GM (to a smaller degree) which have been suppressed by the cytostatic drug [53]. Moreover, while augmenting homing and functional activity of T-lymphocyte that are relatively resistant against the antimetabolite, they simultaneously inhibit recovery of the damaged cells in HIM (assessed by the content and secretory activity of the adherent cells and their ability to form HI based on cell-cell interactions) which disturbs cooperation between the elements of microenvironment in the control of proliferation and differentiation of the progenitor cells resulting in the long-term period of hematopoietic inhibition observed under the action of 5-fluorouracil [40, 53]. Similar uncoupling effect of catecholamines on hematopoiesis was observed under cytostatic treatment with the high doses of cyclophosphane. Such directivity of the influences on the hematopoietic processes was characteristic of glucocorticoids (other family of the stress-mediating hormones) in the animals treated with cytostatic drugs.

By way of conclusion, it should be noted that the changes in hematopoietic control under myelosuppressive influences can be both adaptive and damaging depending on their nature. The accumulated data on the damage exerted by the myeloinhibitory factors of diverse nature at various levels of the blood system and its control apparatus attest to possibility to correct the hematologic pathologies by different ways. The first avenue is based on direct stimulation of proliferation and differentiation of the hematopoietic cells, which is now successfully implemented with various preparations of the hemopoietic growth factors. The second way is to affect the central neuroendocrine hemopoietic control mechanisms with the substances possessing (among other features) the nootropic properties. The third method is to block the peripheral structures responsible for deregulation of the action of the stress-mediating mechanisms on hemopoiesis. Finally, it is visible to modulate the functional activity and structural organization of the local control mechanisms encompassed by the concept of HIM.

Evidently, to implement the above ways to treat the hemopoietic depressions of diverse genesis, it is vitally important to develop the differentiated therapeutic methods.

Chapter 5
Disturbances in Hematopoietic Control During Experimental Leucosis

The modern achievements in pharmacology, genetics, virology, cytology, immunology, and biochemistry paved the way for numerous discoveries in the study of leucosis at the cellular and molecular level. However, no unequivocal solution to the problem of the causes and the developmental mechanisms of this disease has been suggested. The generally accepted theory assumes that some leucosogenic agent can affect a single hemopoietic progenitor cell, which is viewed as the trigger mechanism to form the clone of leukemic cells. Further development of the disease is determined by genetics and mutations. The chromosomal instability which is intrinsic feature of a pathological clone is manifested by repeated mutations leading to formation of malignant clones and tumor progression.

Recent decades are marked with pronounced increase in the research activity focused on the stress effects on the neoplastic processes. The fundamental studies carried out in 1970–1980 taxonomized the stress states that caused tumor growth and examined the peculiarities of psychosocial profile of the oncologic patients to identify the high risk groups and to improve the prevention and treatment methods. It was found that extreme stress reactions are manifested at the long terms in the development of the tumor growth aggravating the somatovisceral and psychoemotional abnormalities. However, the researchers paid little attention to the fact that the clinical stage of any tumor disease is always preceded by the latent period when the pool of malignant cells exists in an organism but does not display the overt signs of the neoplastic process. In this respect, taxonomy of the changes occurring in an organism during the period preceding the evident development of a tumor is of great interest as a tool for early diagnostics and a key in the search for novel methods to prevent and treat the malignant neoplasms.

Spontaneous leucosis in AKR/JY mice is views as a model of human T-cell lympholeucosis. The development of spontaneous leucoses in these mice is genetically determined to result from the vertical transmission of Gross virus. The primary targets for infectious agents are the microenvironment cells in the thymus [288], while the contact of potentially leukemic cells with the stromal elements is a prerequisite condition for triggering the disease [333]. The potentially tumor cells are first

© Springer International Publishing Switzerland 2014
A.M. Dygai, V.V. Zhdanov, *Theory of Hematopoiesis Control*,
SpringerBriefs in Cell Biology 5, DOI 10.1007/978-3-319-08584-5_5

detected in the bone marrow; thereafter they migrate to thymus to be transformed into malignant cells [271]. In the following, the signs of disturbance of medullar hemopoiesis and involvement of the visceral organs into the oncological process are observed.

As early as 1960s, based on the comparative study of normal status of mice with high (AKR/JY) and low (C3H) leukemia incidence, D. Metcalf concluded that the hormonal balance in AKR/JY mice is disturbed. In these mice, production of adrenocortical hormones and sex steroids (the hormones inhibiting lymphocyte proliferation) was down-regulated. As a result, the reproduction of lymphocytes was enhanced resulting in greater size of thymus and other lymphoid organs in AKR/JY mice in comparison to other murine strains. In AKR/JY mice, the mitotic activity of the lymphoid cells in thymus is 6–10 times greater than that in other lymphoid organs being 2 times greater than the activity of lymphoid thymocytes in C3H mice characterized with low leukemia incidence. These peculiarities of mice with high leukemia incidence promote hyperintensive proliferation of thymus cells manifested by thymus hyperplasia needed for leukemogenesis [319]. Our studies showed that young AKR/JY mice had primed erythroid lineage in the bone marrow, while the content of medullar granulocyte-monocyte progenitors and CSA in supernatants harvested from myelocaryocytes were significantly smaller than those of reference CBA/CaLac mice.

Literature describes the stressful influence of infectious agents [78] and tumor process on an organism [7]. In relation to this problem, we examined the state of sympathoadrenal system in AKR/JY mice with high leukemia incidence. The study showed that the dynamics of catecholamine concentration in adrenal medulla is wave-like, although it was decreased during entire examination period in comparison with 2-month CBA/CaLac mice. Partial depletion of the adrenal catecholamines is a characteristic feature of stress reaction, which is observed, in particular, during immobilization stress. In addition, a decrease in the thymus weight at the age of 4–6 months and an increase in total count of myelocaryocytes observed in the aging dynamics of AKR/JY mice also belong to the complex of alterations, which is characteristic of the stress reaction [51, 53].

Our data suggested that aging of AKR/JY mice is accompanied by the development of general adaptation syndrome probably related to circulation of leucosogenic virus in the experimental mice capable to provoke unspecific (adaptive) immune reactions and neoplastic processes. Correspondingly, we conventionally subdivided the changes in the blood system parameters observed in AKR/JY mice during preleucosis period into three interrelated groups: (1) adaptive changes; (2) alterations related to immune reactions against viral antigen; and (3) abnormalities caused by the progress of leucosis.

At the age of 4 months, AKR/JY mice demonstrated a complex of alterations in the blood system, which by many parameters was characteristic of the alarm reaction as a part of general adaptation syndrome provoked by unspecific stimulant in mice with low leucosis incidence [51]. At this age, the above alterations can be related to the spread of leukovirus produced by thymic cells over entire organism.

Of interest are the sex differences in the intensity of alarm reaction within the context of general adaptation syndrome in experimental (AKR/JY) and reference F1(CBA/CaLac*AKR/JY) mice. In females, the hormonal component (depletion of adrenal medulla) is more pronounced, while in the males the blood system adapts to the current stimulant, the adaptation being manifested by more pronounced neutrophilosis, lympho- and eosinopenia in the peripheral blood, and activation of medullar neutrophilopoiesis ranging from the committed to mature forms (bypassing, however, the stage of immature neutrophilic granulocytes). At the same time, the medullar score of granulocyte precursors (CFU-G) in AKR/JY females is significantly decreased probably due to prevalence of the differentiation processes, which limits the potency of granulocytopoiesis. In addition, the females demonstrate prevalence of the signs of hemopoietic cell degeneration related to up-regulation of the apoptotic and necrotic processes. According to our views, responsiveness of the blood system at the 4-month age can be of importance in the mechanisms of lymphogenesis, because decreased incidence of tumor diseases in the males resulting from the effects of androgens [305] is firmly established.

Priming of neutrophilic lineage in 4-month AKR/JY mice (resulting probably from the adaptive and to a lesser degree from the immune processes) is going on against the background of the early degenerative alterations in the erythron. The latter are related to drop in the score of erythroid precursors and erythroid islets in the bone marrow (Fig. 5.1), decrease in the share of erythroid cells in the spleen, and an increase in the score of erythrocytes with micronuclei in the peripheral blood.

It is an established fact that stressful stimulation promotes the release of glucocorticoids from adrenal cortex, which indirectly (via the system of T-lymphocytes) activate all hemopoietic lineages in the bone marrow and the spleen [41]. The 4-month AKR/JY mice are characterized with progressive decrease of metabolic activity of the lymphocytes and down-regulation of IL-1 and IL-2 production to the state of complete arrest accompanied with disturbances in the functional activity of MPS cells [216] which probably leads to abnormalities in erythroid hemopoiesis. At the same time, the thymic lymphoid cells and the lymphatic nodes exert the direct inhibitory effect on hematopoiesis (the erythroid lineage included) at the early stages of tumor development [185].

To the 5–6 months of life, the preleukemic state of AKR/JY mice are characterized with the development of hyperplasia of medullar hemopoiesis attesting to the beginning of the phase of resistance against diverse extreme stimuli [53]. The changes in the blood system parameters probably related to the immune reactions corroborate this reasoning to a certain degree. At this, there is a dramatic activation of granulocytopoiesis mechanisms (increase in the count of precursors and CSA islets, as well as up-regulation of CSA production) accompanied by an increase in the count of mature and immature neutrophilic granulocytes in the bone marrow and elevation of the content of neutrophils in the peripheral blood. However, there is accumulation of CFU-E in the medullar hemopoietic tissue related to up-regulation of functional activity in the cells of hemopoietic microenvironment accompanied by decreased erythropoietic indices according to myelo- and splenograms (Fig. 5.2).

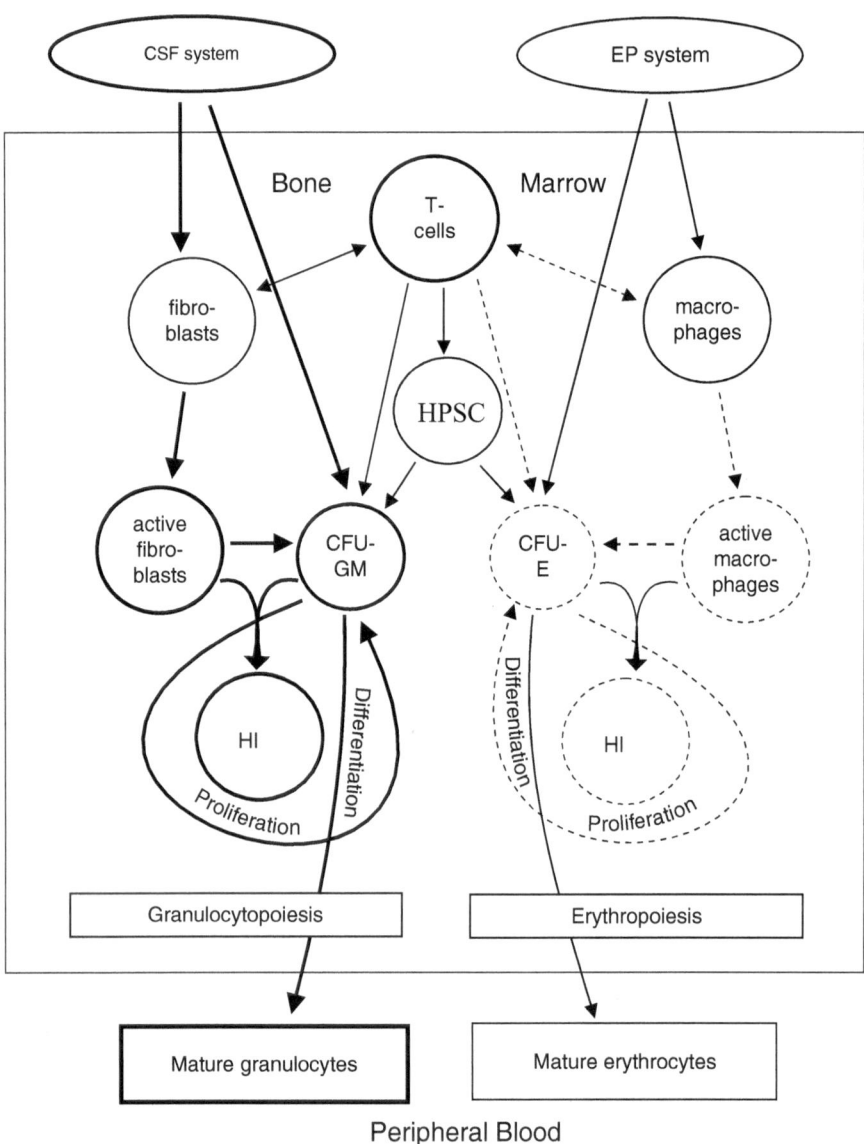

Fig. 5.1 Control of hematopoiesis in 4-month AKR/JY mice. Absence of any significant changes is marked with fine continuous lines, while the *dash* and *thick solid lines* indicate inhibition and activation, correspondingly

In other words, this period of AKR/JY mice life is characterized with limitation of the differentiation potency of the erythroid precursors [31].

The bone marrow of AKR/JY mice contains an enhanced number of the cells with morphology of monoblasts; in addition, there is a certain shift in the ratio of

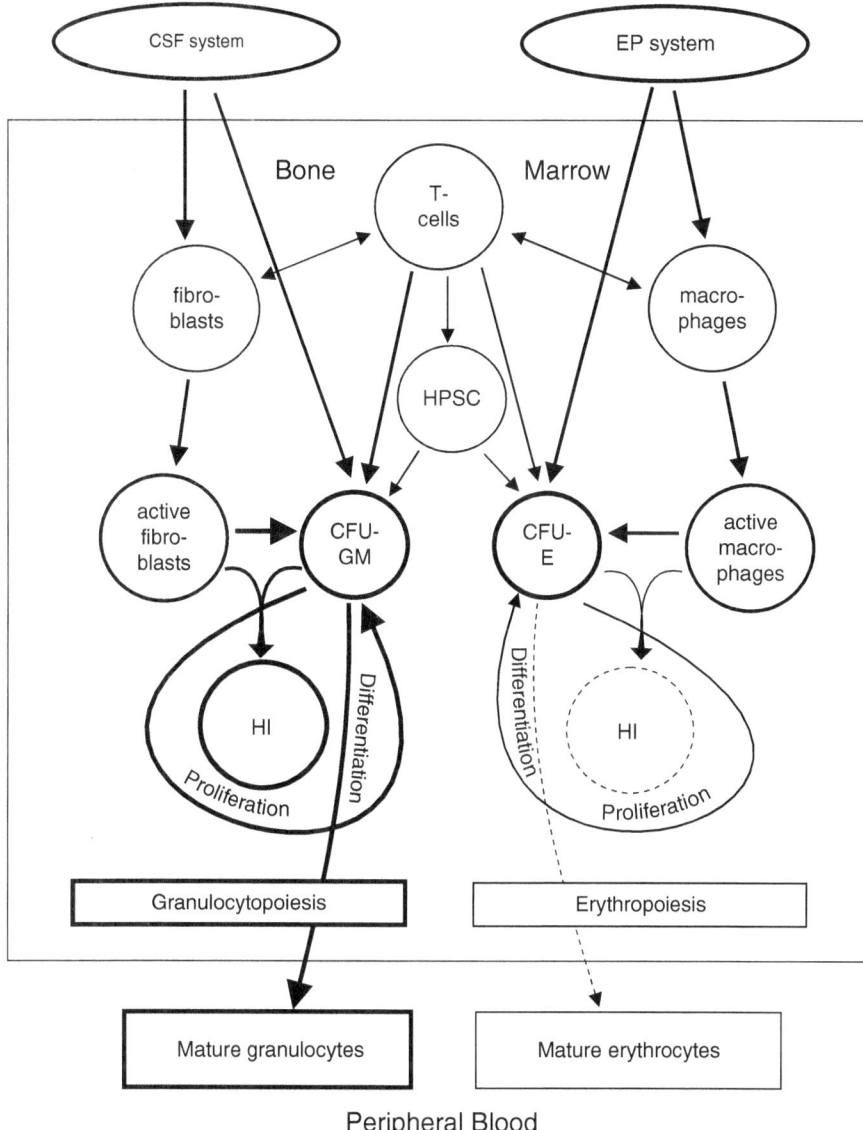

Fig. 5.2 Control of hematopoiesis in 5-month AKR/JY mice. Absence of any significant changes is marked with fine continuous lines, while the *dash* and *thick solid lines* indicate inhibition and activation, correspondingly

stained to non-stained HI in favor of the latter, whose central elements are the immature stromal cells. As the early expression and production of leukoviruses by the stromal cells in AKR/JY mice are the established facts [288], one can expect some structural implementation of the defective hemopoietic microenvironment inducing abnormal hemopoiesis, which is the core of the pathological conceptions such as preleukemia and myelodysplastic syndrome [30, 173].

The development of basic disease in AKR/JY mice with high leucosis incidence provoking the changes of hemopoietic properties of HIM underlies the gradual development of the stage of exhaustion of the processes triggered by the general adaptation syndrome accompanied by the secondary release of catecholamines from adrenal cortex. Unfortunately, the hematological features of this stage were little studied. However, in the cases of hematosarcomas, it is difficult to distinguish them from the alterations caused by the tumor growth. Despite the signs of adaptation syndrome, there was a dramatic aggravation in the general state of 7-month-old AKR/JY mice. The study of blood system revealed the development of lymphoma in 17 % cases, which was accompanied by depletion of the bone marrow (down to 43 % in comparison with healthy animals of the same line) and enhanced leukocytosis in the peripheral blood. Insignificant (about 8 %) replacement of the hemopoietic tissue in the bone marrow with lymphoblasts could be related to pronounced content of the hemopoietic precursors known to possess intrinsic suppressor activity directed to the normal and tumor cells [120]. The following course of events includes probably a drop in the score of the committed progenitor cells due to down-regulation of production of hemopoietins by HIM elements. For instance, in the culture media with low content of stimulants (serum from anemized rabbits or supernatant harvested from the splenocytes), the expansion of CFU-E and precursors of granulomonocytopoiesis (CFU-GM) in 7-month-old mice was markedly inhibited.

On the other hand, the exhaustion phase of AKR/JY mice was characterized with significant increase of the content of fibroblast precursors (CFU-F) as a compensatory reaction to depletion of the bone marrow. Really, there was a drop in the counts of total myelocaryocytes, total blasts, immature and mature forms of neutrophilic granulocytes, as well as erythroid and reticular cells. At this, the changes related to the granulocytic lineage were probably caused by an accelerated release of the cells into peripheral blood. The accelerated granulocytic differentiation was observed in the pool of committed hemopoietic precursors. Really, the CFU-G/CFU-GM ratios in 7-month-old AKR/JY mice, 7-month-old F1(CBA/CaLac*AKR/JY) mice, and 2-month-old CBA/CaLac mice were 44:1, 17:1, and 6:1, respectively. However, a dramatic decrease in the content of MPS cells capable to form granulocyte HI limits the potency of precursors to compensate for the redistributive losses of the granulocytic lineage [29, 173].

At the same time, accumulation of CFU-E in the bone marrow was related to the disturbances in their differentiation caused by decrease in the content of erythroid HI, which in its turn led to a decrease in the number of erythroid mitoses and erythrocaryocytes in the bone marrow. Thus, a drastic inhibition of formation of all HI types resulting from the changes of the properties of the resident macrophages is the pathogenic focus of overall pathologic influence exerted by the neoplastic process on the medullar hemopoiesis in 7-month-old AKR/JY mice with a high leucosis incidence (Fig. 5.3).

The important factors shaping the stress reaction are the genetically determined and acquired peculiarities of an organism (in this respect, the species-related and

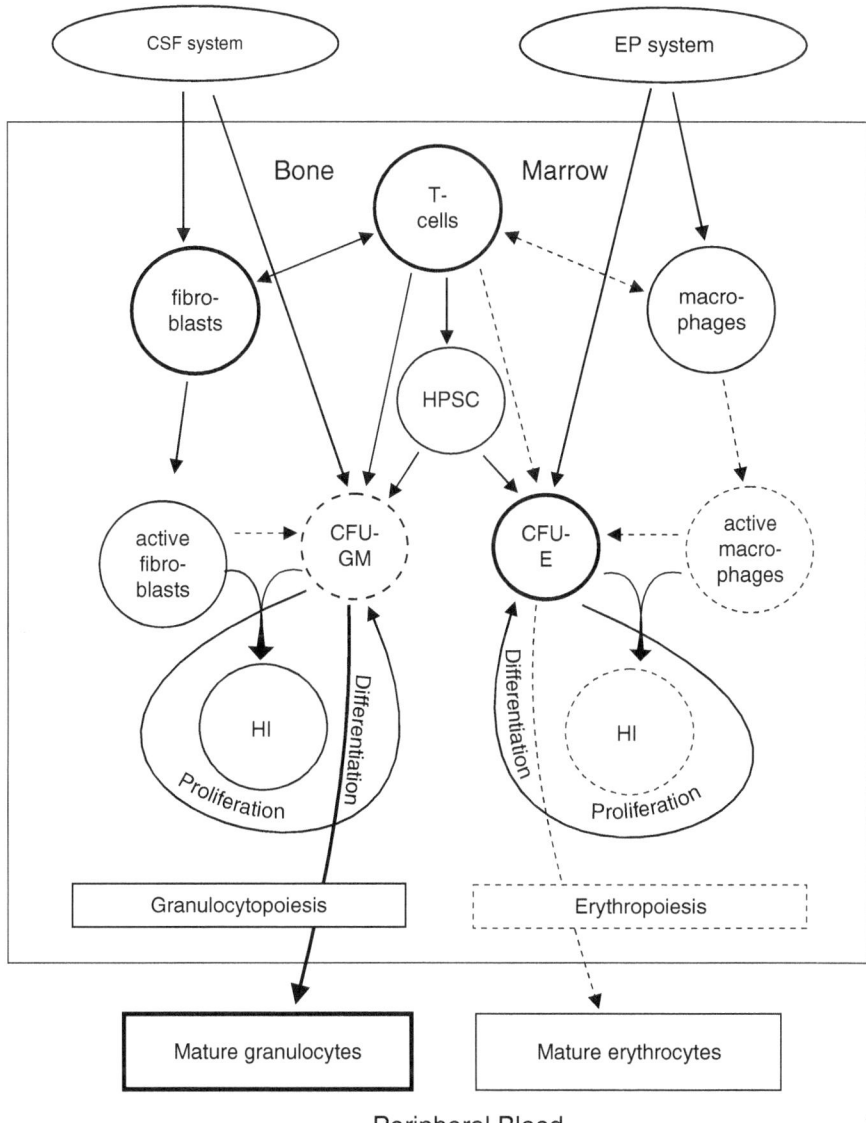

Fig. 5.3 Control of hematopoiesis in 7-month AKR/JY mice. Absence of any significant changes is marked with fine continuous lines, while the *dash* and *thick solid lines* indicate inhibition and activation, correspondingly

typological features of the experimental lines of animals are highly employed in the research work), as well as the state of the organism during the stressful stimulation. The development of adaptive changes under the chronic stress caused by neoplasm growth results in degradation of the stress-mediating systems, which leads not only to inhibition of the general adaptive mechanisms, but also the specific mechanisms of antitumor defense [7]. In this context, we tried to assess the reaction of the blood and sympathoadrenal systems to immobilization stress in AKR/JY mice aging 4 and 7 months to delineate its peculiarities characteristic of this high leukemic line in comparison with F1(CBA/CaLac*AKR/JY) hybrid mice.

The period lasting from day 4 to day 8 after the onset of 6–10 h immobilization is characterized by the development of hyperplasia of the bone marrow. During this period, the hemopoietic tissue displays up-regulation of proliferation, differentiation and migration of the hemopoietic cells [81]. In mice, the stressful stimulation of indicated duration provokes the development of resistance stage of the general adaptation syndrome accompanied by activation of ANS and blood system [51].

Reaction to immobilization of 4-month-old AKR/JY mice was not adequate and commensurable to this stressful stimulation. In contrast to hybrid mice, the mice of high leukemic line demonstrated a dramatic increase in thymus weight and elevation of catecholamines to experiment day 6, which was accompanied by accumulation of the blast cells in thymic tissue and up-regulation of mitotic activity of the lymphocytes. Probably, these changes were related to activation of the pathologic processes in mice organism. An important feature was a drop of total cellularity in the peripheral blood in response to stress accompanied by a decrease in the count of lymphoid cells in the myelogram, which did not agree with the data obtained under similar experimental conditions in mice of low leukemic lines. A decrease in the total number of leukocytes resulted mainly from the drop in the count of lymphoid cells in the peripheral blood. One can hypothesize that glucocorticoids augment the release of lymphocytes from the peripheral blood and their destruction in the reticuloendothelial network accompanied by deposition of the decay products in liver and spleen.

The studies showed that 4-month-old AKR/JY mice react to immobilization with dramatic decrease (down to 45–63 % initial value) in the count of HI with functionally mature stromal elements with the corresponding increase in neutral red staining. At the same time, the content of such elements increased on experiment day 4 in the hybrid mice. In these mice, similar changes in the granulocyte HI count were even more pronounced in comparison with initial level and the corresponding value in stressed AKR/JY mice. At present, involvement of HI in maintaining proliferation and differentiation of hemopoietic precursors from the committed to mature forms is firmly established [51]. It is a known fact that a 10-h immobilization stress up-regulates granulocytopoiesis on days 4–8 of the experiment due to enhancement of proliferative activity and elevation in the count of CFU-GM and HI in murine bone marrow [81]. In our studies, the post-stress drop in the count of granulocyte HI in AKR/JY mice was paralleled by a decrease in the count of CFU-GM in bone marrow, which was especially pronounced on day 4 after the onset of immobilization. In contrast, the initial decrease in the count of CFU-GM in hybrid mice was followed by more than 2-fold elevation of this index in comparison with intact mice or AKR/JY mice exposed to immobilization stress. It is of importance that stress-induced up-regulation of granulocyte HI and CFU-GM formation in F1(CBA/CaLac*AKR/JY) mice was accompanied by hyperplasia of monocytic and granulocytic lineages in the bone marrow related to significant increase in the counts of monocytes (by more than 3 times) as well as immature and mature forms of neutrophil granulocytes (by 1.5 and 2 times, correspondingly). In other words, reaction of granulocytic lineage of medullar hematopoiesis to stress in hybrid F1(CBA/CaLac*AKR/JY) mice is rather balanced, and it virtually does not differ from that of low leukemia mice demonstrating up-regulation of proliferation and differentiation of the committed precursors in HI.

On day 6 after the onset of immobilization, the 4-month-old AKR/JY mice demonstrated increased medullar count of only mature neutrophils. Taking into consideration a decreased count of CFU-GM and granulocytic HI, this fact can indirectly attest to possibility of granulocyte differentiation without concomitant up-regulation of the proliferative activity of the committed precursors.

The data obtained conclude that a limited reaction of the medullar granulocytic lineage provoked by stress in AKR/JY mice is observed as early as life month 4, and it is generally viewed as one of the initial stages of the preleucosis period. This reaction results from disturbances in structure-functional adaptation mechanisms of the hematopoietic tissue to stressful stimulation due to the changes (probably caused by the development of compensatory and adaptive processes) in the hemopoietic properties of the medullar macrophages, which generally agree with the data obtained by M. Hellebostad et al. [272]. The changes in some parameters of functional activity of MPS cells in 4-month-old AKR/JY mice in comparison with 1-month-old mice was reported in the paper of B. Burek and I. Hrsak [216], which can be somewhat related to the early expression of murine leukoviruses by the macrophages observed by S.Y. Kim et al. [288]. On the other hand, the inadequate response of the hematopoietic tissue to the test stressor stimulation attests to imbalance of the distant (first of all, neurohumoral) regulator systems in AKR/JY mice. Really, the 4-month-old AKR/JY mice demonstrate initially pronounced activation of the sympathoadrenal system which exhausts its ability to react to an extra stressful stimulation. Involvement of the sympathoadrenal system into stimulation of granulocytopoiesis is an established fact [51], so limitation of ability of the granulocytic lineage of bone marrow in AKR/JY mice can be explained by enhanced sympathetic tone.

Thus, the initial imbalance between inhibition and activation of the short-range (the cell-cell interaction) and distant (the sympathoadrenal system) regulator mechanisms in 4-month-old AKR/JY mice degrades efficiency of the structure-functional apparatus of granulocytopoiesis resulting in disadaptation of the medullar granulocytic lineage to external stressful load. Probably, in addition to direct involvement of MPS cells in expression and production of leukoviruses, these processes can constitute one of the stages and form one of the pathogenetic mechanisms underlying progression of the lymphoid neoplasia in AKR/JY mice.

By aging, the AKR/JY mice demonstrated the alterations resulted both from the action of specific stimulus (leucosogenic virus) and from the development of general adaptation syndrome. Exposure of 7-month-old high leukemic and hybrid mice to stress resulted in accumulation of CFU-E in the bone marrow (to 129 and 172 % initial levels, correspondingly). However, this accumulation was not accompanied by an increased count of erythrocaryocytes in the hematopoietic tissue. Similar reaction of the erythron to immobilization stress was observed in 4-month-old mice. In this respect, an important feature was a diminished potency of the differentiated erythroid cells of the old mice to proliferate *in vitro* in response to elevated erythropoietin doses that, however, did not change the CFU-E response [365]. Probably, the considered data attest to acceleration of aging processes in AKR/JY mice in comparison with F1(CBA/CaLac*AKR/JY) mice due to earlier manifestation of the disease (month 7 in contrast to month 24 in the hybrid mice). At this, in contrast to 4-month-old mice, degradation of the compensatory potencies in 7-month-old mice affects not only the morphologically resolved elements, but also the pool of the committed erythropoietic progenitors.

In addition, the bone marrow of old AKR/JY mice was characterized by limitation of the functional reserve of the progenitors of granulocytes, macrophages, and the fibroblasts. The count of medullar CFU-GM in intact 7-month-old AKR/JY mice was negligibly larger than that in hybrid mice of the same age and did not significantly differ from this index in 2-month-old CBA/CaLac mice, while the counts of CFU-G and CFU-F were far greater. Probably, a marked increase in CFU-F count reflects the age-dependent changes related to down-regulation of bone marrow hematopoiesis. The immobilization stress pronouncedly down-regulated the colony formation in the culture stimulated with spleen supernatant or recombinant G-CSF. To experiment day 6, the development of CFU-GM, CFU-G, and CFU-F decreased by 1.5–7, 1.5–2, and 1.5–3.5, correspondingly. The hybrid mice demonstrated a pronounced up-regulation of the colony forming processes without stimulation of neutrophilopoiesis and monocytopoiesis in the bone marrow. In both experimental groups, the myelogram revealed a significant increase in the percentage of only mature neutrophilic granulocytes as compared to the initial level. In addition, AKR/JY mice were characterized with the post-stress neutrophilosis in the peripheral blood.

In the same observation period, AKR/JY mice responded to immobilization stress with more than 2-fold drop in the count of all HI forms in the bone marrow, which was initially lower than that in the age-matched hybrid mice. This drop resulted mostly from a decrease in the counts of granulocytic and mixed forms of HI. Decrease in the count of CFU-G and CFU-F to experiment day 6 as well as a drop in the count of CSA and EPA in the supernatants harvested form the cells of unfractionated bone marrow attested to profound alterations in the structure-functional interrelations between the committed precursors and the stromal cells in the bone marrow of old AKR/JY mice. It is most probable that reduction in the count of medullar CFU-GM in AKR/JY mice during the late preleucosis period is underlain by their enhanced granulocytic differentiation from the committed to mature forms which is up-regulated after stressful stimulation. Infection of mouse bone marrow with murine leukemia virus increased the count of the colonies in the granulocytic lineage [258]. However, in contrast to hybrid mice, the 7-month-old AKR/JY mice displayed depletion of functional reserves of granulocytopoiesis which impeded them to respond to an extra stressful stimulation by increasing the pool of committed precursors.

Thus, the late preleucosis period (7th month of life) in AKR/JY mice is probably characterized with restriction of the reserves for proliferation (CFU-GM, CFU-G, CFU-F) and differentiation (CFU-E) of the committed hemopoietic precursors, which makes it impossible to resist stress with an adequate stimulation and expansion of hematopoiesis. However, the reference 7-month-old F1(CBA/CaLac*AKR/JY) hybrid mice display many similar features in the changes of medullar hemopoiesis which can be considered as an earlier stage of the leukemia progression.

Of profound interest is the fact that independent on the mouse age, the counts of apoptotic cells and bodies were significantly higher in AKR/JY mice than in the hybrid ones. It is a common knowledge that apoptosis plays a key role in the control of regeneration of the cell populations [308]. A greater index of the programmed death of the bone marrow cells in high leukemic mice in comparison with the hybrid ones can be related to the development of general adaptation syndrome [368] and the pathologic process.

Immobilization stress significantly decreases both relative and absolute number of apoptotic cells in AKR/JY mice. By contrast, the hybrid mice response to such stress with activation of apoptotic death to experiment day 4 after immobilization and with recovery of the apoptotic index up to initial level to experiment day 6.

The data attest to profound abnormalities in the mechanisms of cellular self-regulation manifested in AKR/JY mice as early as the fourth month of life. Taking into consideration the fact that the bone marrow of sick 10-month-old mice of this line contains a large number (up to 9 %) of actively phagocytizing macrophages, one can hypothesize that the apoptotic death of the myelocaryocytes is one of the reasons of depletion of the hematopoietic tissue characteristic of lymphoma development.

Thus, during the period of life of the high leukemic AKR/YJ mice encompassing 4–7 months defined as preleucosis, a number of signs are manifested that suggest the development of general adaptation syndrome. There are two critical periods in aging dynamics of these mice. The first period (at the age of 4 months) relates probably to active expression of the viral agent. It is characterized with intensive maturation of the elements of granulocytic lineage of hematopoiesis accompanied by inhibition of erythropoiesis. These peculiarities are revealed most clearly after a 10-h immobilization used as a test stressful load. At the age of 5–6 months, an organism mobilizes the compensatory mechanisms resulting in hyperplasia of the bone marrow. At this period, the imbalance of structural organization of hemopoiesis is manifested more clearly. Finally, the compensatory potencies of the blood system are exhausted to the age of 7 months resulting in persistent decrease of hemopoietic potency accompanied with alterations in the peripheral hemopoiesis. Probably, this state precedes manifestations of the clinical symptoms of leucosis.

Chapter 6
Disturbances in the Control of Blood System During Posthypoxic Period

One of the pivotal problems in experimental and clinical medicine is adaptation to hypoxia. Almost any pathologic process is more or less accompanied with the development of a particular type of hypoxia. The hypoxic stimulation exerts a powerful effect on the transport of blood gases resulting in the functional and then the structural rearrangements in the mechanisms supplying oxygen for an organism. On the whole, these changes sustain the energy metabolism [1, 10, 14, 124, 126, 147, 159, 235].

The changes evolving in the peripheral blood and in the bone marrow during hypoxic stimulation are described in detail [14, 108, 121, 133, 196, 198, 268]. Generally, the blood system reacts to hypoxia with an increase of oxygen capacity by increasing the number of erythrocytes and elevating the hemoglobin content. These adaptive changes results from the reflex release of the mature cells from depot as well as from activation and increase in the count of erythroid lineage in the hemopoietic organs [14, 109, 142, 198]. In its turn, activation of erythropoiesis results from elevation of the count of HSC in the bone marrow and peripheral blood [178, 201, 214, 222, 275, 321, 360], as well as from up-regulation of erythropoietin (erythrogenin) production by the renal juxtamerular apparatus [142, 175, 198, 236]. As a rule, these processes are accompanied with the development of leukocytosis in the peripheral blood (mostly of lymphocytic type) which is explained by migration of T-lymphocytes known as the regulators of hemopoiesis into hematopoietic tissue [53, 198]. In the early terms after exposure to hypoxia, neutrophilosis is less often observed, and it is viewed as a manifestation of the general adaptation syndrome [53, 154–156, 175, 196].

Irrespective to its cause, hypoxia is always accompanied by the development of unidirectional reactions in the hematopoietic tissue. However, the mode and length of hypoxic stimulation can determine many features of the specific changes formed at various organization strata of the blood system. We carried out a comprehensive study of the role of individual elements in HIM and that of the distant neurohumoral hemopoietic control mechanisms during hypoxia of various genesis and severity [43, 101–105].

© Springer International Publishing Switzerland 2014   59
A.M. Dygai, V.V. Zhdanov, *Theory of Hematopoiesis Control*,
SpringerBriefs in Cell Biology 5, DOI 10.1007/978-3-319-08584-5_6

The experiments were conducted on CBA/CaLac mice. The experimental model were based on hypoxic-hypercapnic normobaric hypoxia (hypoxic hypoxia) and two variants of hemic hypoxia, which developed under (1) hemolytic or (2) post-hemorrhagic anemia. The hypoxic hypoxia was simulated with single or double (10 min prior to the second exposure) placing the mice in a 500-ml hermetic chamber. The hemic hypoxia was modeled either with intraperitoneal injection of phenylhydrazine hydrochloride (30 or 150 mg/kg) or puncture of retro-orbital sinus for blood withdrawal (30 % circulation blood volume in a single procedure or 70 % with triple bleedings performed during 2–3 h). The intact mice were used to obtain the control indices.

A single exposure to hypoxia in the hermetic chamber, injection of the hemolytic toxin (30 mg/kg), or withdrawal 30 % circulating blood (volume percentage) produced no significant changes in the psychoneurological status. Severe oxygen deficiency (double hypoxia in the hermetic chamber, injection of 150 mg/kg hemo-lytic toxin, or withdrawal 70 % circulating blood) provoked the encephalopathia documented according to the development of amnesia assessed according to the disturbances in the conditioned passive avoidance test and in orienting-exploratory behavior tested in the 'open field' environment [13, 369].

The experiments showed that hypoxia of various geneses that provoked no 'overt' disorders in the psychoneurological status induced a pronounced hyper-plasia of the erythroid hemopoietic lineage. During the entire period of such experiments, there was a pronounced elevation of the erythrocaryocyte count in hematopoietic tissue, which was especially great during hypoxic hypoxia (up to 438.8 % baseline on experiment day 5). Activation of the medullar erythropoiesis was echoed in the peripheral blood by elevation in the reticulocyte count observed on days 1–3, 5, 8 and 9 after hypoxic hypoxia and during the entire observation period under any type of hemic hypoxia attaining the maximum level on day 10 after injection of the hemolytic toxin (671.5 % baseline value). The changes in erythrocyte content were mostly determined by specificity of hypoxic stimula-tion; they were characterized by the drop in erythrocyte count coupled with decreased hematocrit after withdrawal 30 % circulation blood (days 1–5) or injection of phenylhydrazine (days 1–10). In contrast, hypoxic hypoxia induced erythrocytosis developed on experiment days 1–6. The qualitative analysis of the blood formed elements revealed a slight increase in the volume of the mature erythrocytes resulting probably from release of a great number of young erythro-cytes into the circulating blood [26, 98]. However, this index decreased in the early terms of hemolytic anemia (days 1–3). Evidently, this phenomenon resulted from destruction of the largest cells by the toxin during their transport in the microcirculatory bed. In addition to the changes in the size of erythrocytes observed on days 1 and 3 after hemoexfusion, there was elevation of the mean corpuscle content of hemoglobin probably related to the fact that a pronounced share of hematocrit was comprised by the erythrocytes released from the depot. Formation of these erythrocytes was going on under the conditions of balanced hemopoiesis characterized by a rather high activity of the hemoglobin-producing processes and a rather low maturation rate of erythroid precursors. Moreover, all three groups displayed a decreased osmotic resistance of erythrocytes, which attained the minimum level on day 1 after injection of the hemolytic toxin.

As for granulocytopoiesis, any model of hypoxia was characterized with different increase in the count of immature and mature neutrophilic granulocytes in hematopoietic tissue, which attained the maximum values in the blood loss hypoxia model. This phenomenon was accompanied with increase in the count of the rod neutrophils in peripheral blood.

The described changes in hematopoiesis were preceded by up-regulation of the colony-forming potency of the bone marrow. Irrespective of its mode, hypoxia was accompanied with increase in formation of CFU-E and CFU-GM in the methyl cellulose medium. In all cases, the proliferative activity of the committed precursors of both types increased, and maturation of erythroid precursors accelerated virtually during entire period of examination. In addition, differentiation of the precursor cells of granulomonocytopoiesis was up-regulated after hemic hypoxia (hemolytic anemia), while it was down-regulated after hypoxic hypoxia.

The state of the pool of clonogenic cells is known to be mainly determined by the level of production of a wide spectrum of the humoral hemopoietic regulators (first of all, the hemopoietic growth factors) by the cellular components in HIM [37, 255]. Among the hormone-like agents, these growth factors are the most powerful hemopoietic regulators [57, 134, 299], and their combined effect can be assessed as EPA and CSA [56].

The study of secretion activity of some bone marrow fractions under various types of hypoxia showed an increase of EPA in the conditioned media harvested from the adherent and non-adherent nucleated cells in all groups and virtually at any term of examination. Elevation of CSA in the supernatants harvested from the adherent elements was observed during various terms of experiments under hypoxic hypoxia, hemolytic anemia, and after blood loss. It was also observed in the conditioned media of the non-adherent myelocaryocytes after injection of the hemolytic toxin. In contrast, the hypoxic hypoxia and blood loss down-regulated CSA production by the non-adherent fraction of the bone marrow.

The key role in the control of hemopoiesis (especially under the stressful conditions) is played by the serum humoral factors – specifically, the hormones of adrenal cortex and medulla, opioid peptides, eicosanoids, and other endogenous biologically active substances [53, 90, 299]. The experiments showed that irrespective of its type, hypoxia increased serum CSA, which attests to activation of the stress-mediating systems during hypoxia.

However, the development of adaptive reactions in the hematopoietic tissue during oxidative failure of various geneses is mainly determined by enhancement of functional activity of the erythropoietin-producing renal apparatus [26, 349]. It is an established fact that the products of erythrocyte degradation stimulate erythropoiesis [37, 136, 180]. It is also known that hypoxic stimulation activates the processes of erythrodiaeresis.

When studying the role of humoral factors in producing the hypoxia-induced hematological alterations, all the employed models revealed elevation in the contents of erythropoietically active substances in the blood serum. However, while

EPA dynamics was similar in all hypoxia models, the content of erythropoietin significantly differed in these models both in the periods and in the degree of EPA elevation. It is noteworthy that no model displayed a close conformity between EPA dynamics and the erythropoietin content, which shows that erythropoietin does not play any pronounced role in determining the level of total serum EPA.

Really, the up-regulation of colony formation in the test system induced by the serum derived under hypoxic hypoxia was observed on experiment days 1–5, 9, and 10 (attaining maximum 299.7 % baseline value on day 3), while increase in erythropoietin content was recorded in 12 h after hypoxia and on experiment days 1, 2, and 6–9 with the largest value of 363.3 % attained in 12 h after stimulation. In contrast, hemolytic anemia increased EPA in the blood serum, while the blood content of erythropoietin was significantly elevated only on experiment day 7. Hemoexfusion of 30 % circulating blood volume increased serum EPA and the content of serum erythropoietin virtually at the same time: on experiment days 1–3, 7, and 9 (EPA), and in 12 h and on experiment days 1–3 and 9 (erythropoietin). However, these indices significantly differed by the degree of elevation.

In all hypoxia models, the degree of hemolysis greatly increased in the periods when there was no correlation between EPA and the serum level of erythropoietin (on experiment days 3, 5; 1–10; and days 4, 6 after hypoxic hypoxia, hemolytic anemia, and blood loss, correspondingly). This fact indicates a pronounced contribution of the products of erythrocyte degradation into formation of serum EPA.

Investigation of cooperation between various HIM elements and the hemopoietic cells under diverse hypoxia models revealed enhancement of the potency of the supplementary elements in the bone marrow to form the cell associations. Specifically, hypoxic hypoxia increased the count of macrophage-positive and macrophage-negative associations. The qualitative analysis showed elevation in the count of erythroid HI in the hematopoietic tissue on experiment das 2, 3, 5, 6, and 8–10, although the significant elevations in the counts of their mixed and granulocytic types were observed only on days 2 and 3.

Similar alterations in the structure-functional organization of the bone marrow were also observed after hemic hypoxia. Both variants of hemic hypoxia enhanced the adhesive potency of macrophagal elements and the fibroblasts towards the hemopoietic precursors. These changes in activity of the adherent myelocaryocytes were regularly accompanied by a pronounced elevation of the content of erythroid HI in the bone marrow during virtually entire observation period attaining maximum of 386.2 % baseline value on day 7 after injection of hemolytic toxin or 359.0 % on day 5 after hemoexfusion. Elevations in the score of granulocytic and mixed cell associations were far less pronounced.

Taking into consideration the prominent role of lymphoid elements (specifically, Thy-1,2+-cells) in the development of adaptive reactions in the blood system provoked by stressful stimulation [44, 90], we examined activity of these cells in the control of hemopoiesis during hypoxia. The experiments showed that various by their nature stimuli triggered the development of unidirectional changes in the count of Thy-1,2+-cells in the bone marrow. In all cases their number in the hematopoietic tissue significantly increased on experiment days 2–4 after hypoxic hypoxia and on days 1–4 after hemolytic anemia. All hypoxia models revealed a pronounced stimulation of functional activity of hemopoietic precursors under the effect of the above regulator elements accompanied by elevation in the count of medullar T-cells. Especially pronounced were the feeder activity of Thy-1,2$^+$-cells towards the hemo-poietic precursor cells during their interaction with the elements of HIM adherent fraction. It is worthy to note that after hypoxic hypoxia or blood loss, this activating effect was more pronounced in respect to proliferation and differentiation of the erythroid precursors than to those of CFU-GM.

The data obtained proved the important role of T-cells with Thy-1,2$^+$ phenotype in the development of hyperplasia of the hematopoietic tissue during hypoxia of diverse geneses. The research showed that Thy-1,2$^+$-cells exerted the stimulatory effect on the committed erythropoietic precursors both directly and indirectly via interaction with the adherent elements of the bone marrow, while in respect to the granulocyte-macrophage precursors, they displayed the feeder activity only indi-rectly via cooperation with the stromal elements.

An extra mathematical processing of the data with analysis of significant rank correlation coefficients (r) under diverse hypoxic stimulation revealed a marked increase in the number of signal correlations between the individual compartments of erythron system in all employed hypoxia models reflecting a high degree of coupling in the erythropoiesis-stimulating performance of various regulator systems such as HIM or erythropoietin system. In this orchestrated activity, the coordinating role in shaping the response of the hematopoietic tissue is evidently given to the central (neuroendocrine) regulatory subdivision. It is noteworthy that the hemolytic anemia was characterized with a positive correlation between serum EPA and hemolysis. At the same time, the data reduction performed with the factor analysis for any type of hypoxia, revealed the predominant dependence of blood profile on the formation of the extra structure-functional units in the bone marrow, *i.e.* on erythroid HI. However, no hypoxia model displayed any significant changes in the correlation matrix of the data characterizing the processes of granulomonocytopoiesis. The load factor analysis revealed a significant enhancement of serum CSA role in the response of granulomonocytic hemopoietic lineage indicating the growing importance of the long-range humoral mechanisms in the control of granulomonocytopoiesis during various types of hypoxia and under sustaining the initially low coordination level in the performance of individual HIM elements.

Thus, hypoxia of various geneses, which produces no damage to CNS, triggers the development of clearly manifested compensation-adaptation reactions in the blood system such as pronounced hyperplasia of erythroid hemopoietic lineage responsible for the oxygen supply to the tissues and stimulation of granulocytopoiesis reflecting activation of the stress-mediating systems [40]. These alterations are determined by migration of hemopoietic regulator T-cells into the bone marrow, their cooperation with the stromal elements in hematopoietic tissue, enhancement of feeder activity of the cellular components in HID, and elevation of the content of hematopoietically active serum substances. The data obtained attest to profound role of not only erythropoietin, but also other substances in forming serum EPA and conse-quently, in shaping the response of erythron system to hypoxia (Fig. 6.1).

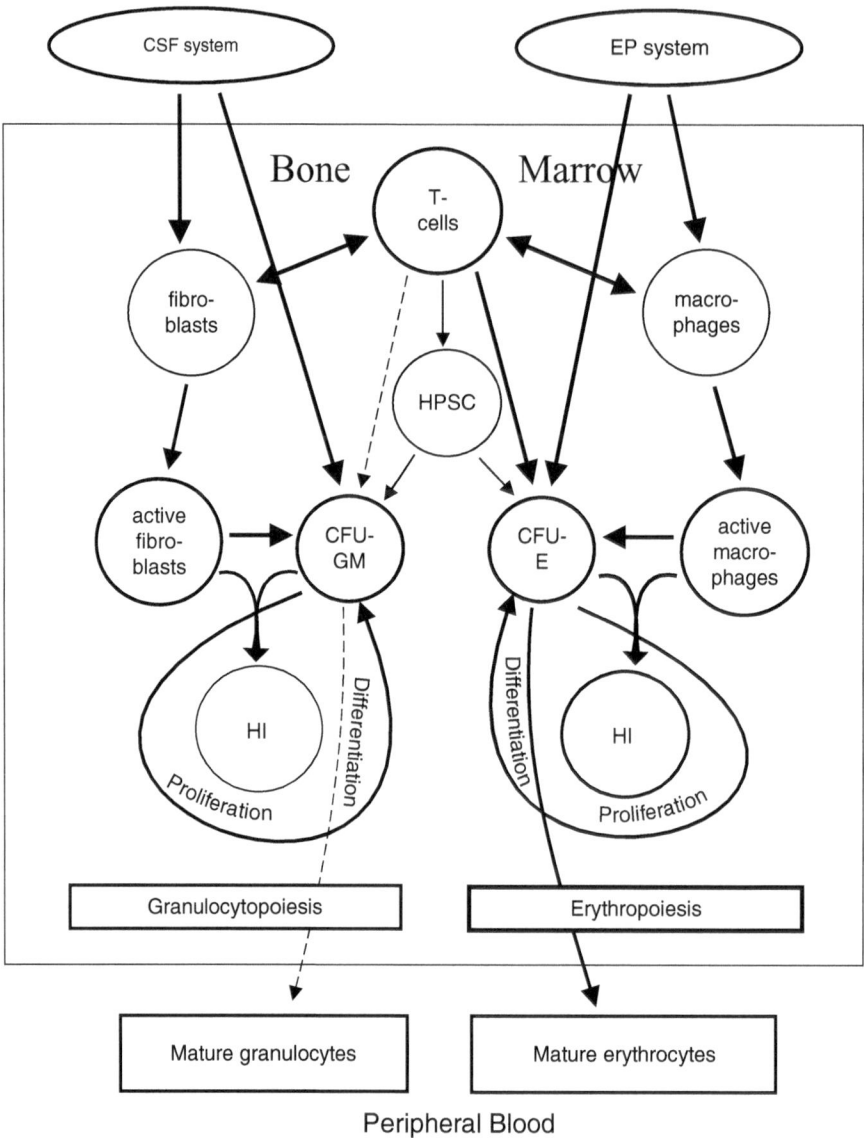

Fig. 6.1 Control of hematopoiesis during mild hypoxia provoking no damage to CNS. Absence of any significant changes is marked with fine continuous lines, while the *dash* and *thick solid lines* indicate inhibition and activation, correspondingly

The comparative analysis of hematological alterations in the employed hypoxia models showed that the most efficient reaction of erythropoiesis was observed under hemic hypoxia. It is explained by a high rate of maturation of the erythroid precursors and rapid release of erythrocytes from the hemopoietic organs. Certain differences were also observed in the reactions of granulomonocytic lineage. In all hypoxia models, intensity of proliferation of hemopoietic precursors increased, which however was not accompanied (or little accompanied) by activation of their differentiation after hypoxic hypoxia and blood loss. Hemolytic anemia did not uncouple these processes, which probably resulted from a high oxygen deficiency during this type of hypoxia and production of a large amount of phlogogenic substances in hypoxia-damaged tissues [96, 303].

However, literature reports that pronounced inhibition of aerobic oxidation in cerebral tissues significantly reorganizes CNS, modifies the integrative-triggering activity of the neurons resulting in a qualitatively novel pattern of interaction of individual cerebral subdivisions. In case of decompensation of the adaptive mechanisms, a chain of pathologic process is triggered leading to progressive neurological disorders and abnormalities in the work of numerous visceral organs and systems [5, 119, 132, 138, 139].

Further stage of our studies was examination of possible influence of encephalopathia as a hematopoiesis-dysregulating process on the formation of hematological alterations during severe hypoxia.

Investigation of the reactions of hematopoietic tissue in animals with hypoxia-induced cerebral pathology revealed a number of interesting features. Irrespective to the triggering cause, encephalopathy was accompanied with a delayed decrease in the level of hyperplasia of hemopoietic lineage resulting from a decrease in the count of hemopoietic precursors and moderation of their proliferative activity. In particular, the hypoxic hypoxia diminished CFU-E content on experiment days 4, 5, 8, and 9, while the count of mitotically active precursors decreased as early as day 1 of experiment. The development of cerebral pathology provoked by hemolytic agent or 70 % blood volume loss was accompanied with a decrease in the colony-forming potency of the bone marrow on, respectively, experiment days 4, 6, 7, 9 or 4, 9 as well as with down-regulation of DNA synthesis in CFU-E observed on days 5–7 (hemolytic anemia) or on days 3, 8, 9 (blood loss) in comparison to the control values measured in the animals without encephalopathy.

In all hypoxia models and during entire observation period, there was a compensatory activation of the processes of CFU-E differentiation related to up-regulation of the secreting function of the adherent myelocaryocytes, elevated serum EPA, accompanied by up-regulation of the formation of the erythroid cell associations after injection of 150 mg/kg phenylhydrazine or extensive blood loss.

Severe hypoxia produced quite equivocal effect on the humoral mechanisms of erythropoiesis control. While after hypoxic hypoxia or blood loss the increase in EPA was greater than elevation of erythropoietin content, the severe hemolysis pronouncedly elevated erythropoietin content almost during entire observation period, but decreased serum EPA at the late terms of experiment. In addition, irrespective to the exciting cause of encephalopathy, all animals with this pathology demonstrated dramatic elevation in the degree of hemolysis.

The study of T-lymphocytic mechanisms of hematopoietic control under severe oxygen deficiency of diverse genesis showed that the development of CNS pathology in all cases led to pronounced and long-term decrease in the count of Thy-1,2$^+$-cells in the bone marrow practically to the level characteristic of the intact animals. At the same time, even a small amount of these cells efficiently stimulated CFU-E in the culture, but this effect was observed only when they interacted with the elements of adherent fraction of myelocaryocytes. These data conclude that preservation of activity of one of the trigger elements of erythropoietic stimulation (T-cells of hematopoietic tissue) during severe hypoxia of various geneses is related not to the changes in the count of medullar population of Thy-1,2$^+$-cells, but to their functional state. However, virtually in all cases with severe encephalopathia, Thy-1,2$^+$-lymphocytes lost the ability to individually affect the proliferation-differentiation status of the erythroid precursors without cooperation with the resident HIM cells.

The changes in examined parameters of granulomonocytic hemopoietic lineage were in many respects similar to the dynamics of erythropoietic indices. Specifically, the medullar count of granulomonocytic progenitors decreased after hypoxic hypoxia (on day 4), hemolytic anemia (on days 2, 4, 5, 7 and 9), and blood loss (days 9–10). In all cases, these changes were preceded by (1) a decrease in CFU-GM division rate, which was most pronounced after injection of 150 mg/kg phenylhydrazine (down to 54.4 % control value on postinjection day 7) and (2) an increase in maturation rate of granulomonocytic precursors. The latter phenomenon resulted from an increased level of CSA in the tested biological fluids. Severe hypoxic stimulation (hypoxic hypoxia) and a high volume of blood loss up-regulated formation of CSA by the adherent and non-adherent nucleated cells of the bone marrow; in addition, it elevated the content of serum hemopoietins after hypoxic hypoxia and posthemorrhagic encephalopathia. In contrast, the development of cerebral pathology provoked by the hemolytic toxin significantly enhanced CSA in the conditioned media of the bone marrow cells without any discernible effect on serum CSA.

However, an increase of hypoxia severity in all cases was accompanied with a marked enhancement of ability of Thy-1,2$^+$-cells to stimulate the growth of granulomonocytic precursors either in the pool of medullar cells cultured on adhesive cell sublayer or (in contrast to hypoxia not accompanied with encephalopathia) in individually cultured non-adherent elements. Efficiency of the influence of these cells on colony formation mediated via their interaction with the adherent myelocaryocytes was pronouncedly greater than that observed during naturally similar hypoxic states that did not disturb the psychoneurological status (especially in the hemolytic variant of hypoxia). Taking into consideration the results of the study, one can conclude that a severe degree of oxygen deficiency determined the following change in the vector of the direct feeder influence of Thy-1,2$^+$-cells from predominant action on erythroid precursors after compensated hypoxia to stimulation of granulomonocytopoiesis after severe hypoxia aggravated with developing encephalopathia.

Despite the same kind of alterations in the state of granulocyte-macrophage precursors and spectacular similarity in the changes of regulatory mechanisms in all hypoxia models, there were significant differences between the experimental groups in the content of morphologically identifiable cells of granulocytic moiety. For example, while massive hemolysis and blood loss decreased the count of immature and mature granulocytes in the bone marrow relative to the baseline values, the hypoxic hypoxia elevated the counts of mature granulocytes on experiment days

3, 7, 8 and 10. In all hypoxia models, we observed the development of neutrophilic leukocytosis in the peripheral blood, which attained the maximum level (up to 437.4 % baseline value on experiment day 1) in the cases with encephalopathia caused by the hemolytic toxin. Probably, this phenomenon resulted not so much from accelerated differentiation of the granulomonocytic precursors, but rather from the disturbances in the efflux of the toxically damaged leucocytes from the tissues [26].

Irrespective to its cause, the damage to CNS was accompanied with the changes in the parameters of peripheral part of the erythron system. The hypoxic animals demonstrated either the development (hypoxic hypoxia) or aggravation of anemia. At the high doses of phenylhydrazine or after a massive blood loss, this anemia was related to specificity of stimulation characterized with the maximum drop in the count of erythrocytes to 35.1 % (day 6) or 54.4 % (day 3) baseline value, correspondingly. In addition, despite the clearly displayed reticulocytic reaction, one of the reasons of anemia was abnormality of the recovery dynamics of erythrocyte content due to the development of macrocytosis and degradation in osmotic resistance of the cells virtually during entire observation period resulting in rapid dieresis of the newly formed large erythrocytes. In the cases with encephalopathia provoked by hypoxic hypoxia, anemia was delayed and hypochromic, which can be probably explained by extreme enlargement of the mature erythrocytes and by a decrease in their hemoglobinization during the overstressed erythropoiesis.

In all encephalopathia models, the correlation and factor analyses revealed a pronounced decrease in the number of causal relationships between the numerical parameters of erythron and the functional activity of the erythropoietic control systems during the changes in the factor loads of the correlation matrix. This fact reflects a diminished role of cell-cell cooperation in mediating the response of the erythron system in contrast to that of serum EPA, which probably attests to dysregulation of hematopoiesis during hypoxia inducing the pathologic changes in CNS. In addition, all cases of severe hypoxia were characterized with a positive correlation between increase of serum EPA and intensity of hemolysis.

However, in the model of phenylhydrazine-induced encephalopathia the mathematical analysis of granulomonocytopoiesis revealed an increase in the number of signal relationships between the individual compartments of granulomonocytic lineage, which attested to enhancement of system stress. In all cases, reduction of the correlation bonds performed with the factor analysis revealed an increasing role of the humoral regulators produced by the stromal HIM components, which in the cases of hypoxic hypoxia and blood loss was also accompanied with decreasing role of serum hemopoietins in shaping the reactions of leucocytes to hypoxia. These facts indicate the changes in the character of granulocytopoiesis control during severe hypoxic stimulation.

Overall, the data obtained make it possible to describe the state of the blood system resulting from failure of the compensation-adaptation hemopoietic mechanisms during hypoxia as a kind of 'erythropoietic distress' manifested by disadaptation of the hematopoietic tissue and production of the pathological forms of erythrocytes.

At this state, the decrease in the count of hematopoietic precursors accompanied with enhancement of functional activity of the relatively resistant stromal components in HIM can be related to their damage due to extreme activation of the sympathoadrenal and pituitary-adrenal systems. As we mentioned in the above, such inverse (negative) effect of surplus of the catecholamines on the hemopoietic precursor cells was observed in the model of cytostatic myelosuppression provoked by antimetabolite injection [53]. As for the pathologic hyperactivity of sympathoadrenal system during hypoxia, it can result from dysfunction of inhibitory mediator systems known for their high sensitivity to oxygen deficiency [5, 132].

To test the hypothesis about the central genesis of the revealed hematologic phenomena in severe hypoxia, the exposed mice were treated with a single intraperitoneal injection of sodium oxybutirate (500 mg/kg), which in all cases eliminated the psychoneurological signs of encephalopathia and significantly corrected the manifestations of disadaptation in the blood system.

The pharmacological protection of the brain elevated the count of progenitor cells in the bone marrow tissue observed in the cases of severe hypoxic hypoxia (experiment days 3–5, 8), toxin-induced hemolysis (day 6), and massive blood loss (day 3). In all cases, these changes were accompanied with increasing proliferative activity of the precursor cells up the levels characteristic of the mice subjected to the milder variants of the corresponding hypoxic stimulation producing no dramatic disturbances in CNS. Logically, the compensation for the disturbances in the committed progenitor cells resulted in hyperplasia of erythroid hemopoietic lineage accompanied by arresting the development of anemia resulted from hypoxic hypoxia. Injection of sodium oxybutirate during severe hemolytic anemia and 70 % blood volume loss was accompanied by an increase in the count of erythrocytes in the peripheral blood. In this case, the size of mature erythrocytes was significantly decreased, which was not accompanied by any significant changes in the release of reticulocytes into the blood.

Examination of secretory function of individual HIM components after neuroprotective treatment and exposure of the mice to severe hypoxia revealed down-regulation of EPA production by the adherent myelocaryocytes on experiment day 4 (hypoxic hypoxia), on days 1, 7, 10 (hemolytic anemia), and on day 7 (massive blood loss). However, injection of sodium oxybutirate produced virtually no effect on (1) feeder activity of Thy-1,2$^+$-cells for CFU-E, (2) production of EPA by non-adherent cells in the bone marrow, and (3) serum EPA. These facts show that during total oxygen deficiency, hemopoiesis is mostly affected by the direct effects of hypoxia on HIM mobile elements (T-cells included) and on the distant humoral mechanisms of hematopoietic control in contrast to indirect effects of hypoxia on hematopoiesis mediated via CNS.

Injection of sodium oxybutirate also elevated the count of granulomonocytopoiesis precursors in the hematopoietic tissue in mice subjected to hypoxic hypoxia, hemolytic anemia, and blood loss, which was accompanied by an increase in their division rate. However, CFU-GM maturation index decreased in all cases. In all groups, the above alterations resulted from down-regulation of CSA production by the adherent medullar nucleated cells, and after hypoxic hypoxia or blood loss they were accompanied by a decrease in the serum content of granulomonocytopoiesis inducers. Nevertheless, intensity of differentiation of the granulomonocytic precursors under the antihypoxant action of sodium oxybutirate significantly surpassed this parameter in animals subjected to the corresponding types of hypoxia that did not provoke lesion to CNS. In all cases, a comparatively high maturation rate of the progenitor cells of granulomonocytopoiesis was related to retention of feeder activity of Thy-1,2$^+$-cells for CFU-GM, up-regulation of CSA production by the non-adherent myelocaryocytes during the early posthypoxic period, and an enhanced level of serum hemopoietins during the late posthypoxic period. Finally, the changes in proliferation-differentiation status of CFU-GM resulted in elevation in the count of mature neutrophilic granulocytes in the bone marrow on experiment days 5, 7 (hemolytic anemia), and on days 3, 4, 6 (blood loss), but they produced no significant effect on the score of morphologically identifiable cells of granulocytopoiesis in the case of hypoxic hypoxia in comparison with the animals not treated with the antihypoxant agent.

In all hypoxia models, the described ambiguous alterations in the medullar granulocytopoiesis in mice treated with sodium oxybutirate were reflected in the peripheral blood by a decrease in the count of segmented neutrophils relatively to the control values as assessed on experiment days (3–7), (1, 2, 6, 7), and (7–9) after hypoxic hypoxia, hemolytic anemia, and blood loss, correspondingly. However, this index remained enhanced in comparison with the corresponding values in the animals exposed to the same types of hypoxia, which did not provoke encephalopathia. In our opinion, maintenance of a high level of neutrophil production is underlain by physiologically reasonable necessity to 'clear' the tissues from detritus [78, 303], whose production is pronouncedly increased with aggravation of hypoxia.

The experimental data unequivocally attest to interrelation between cerebral pathology caused by 'global' hypoxia of diverse geneses with decrease in the number of hemopoietic precursors in the hematopoietic tissue, enhancement of the feeder activity of the stromal components in HIM, and up-regulation of production of the pathological forms of erythrocytes (Fig. 6.2).

Under severe hypoxia, the most probable reason of the alterations in the blood system especially manifested by the disturbances in hematopoiesis is the damage to the hematopoietic cells by the adrenergic overstimulation. In such cases, the effects of catecholamines are predominantly mediated via β-adrenergic receptors [47, 53].

Examination of the role of the adrenergic hemopoietic control mechanisms in shaping the hematological alterations during hypoxia aggravated by encephalopathia showed that blockade of β-adrenergic receptors with a single subcutaneous injection of propranolol (5 mg/kg) made after double hypoxic hypoxia elevated the count of erythrocytes in the peripheral blood (experiment days 4, 7, 9), increased the hemoglobin content (day 5), and abrogated the development of hypochromic anemia in posthypoxic period. Moreover, propranolol markedly improved the recovery dynamics of erythrocyte indices in the cases of severe hemolytic and hemorrhagic anemia. In the cases of hemic hypoxia caused by phenylhydrazine (150 mg/kg) and hemorrhagic anemia provoked by massive blood loss, the count of erythrocytes was elevated correspondingly on experiment days 6–9 and 5, 6, 9, while hematocrit increased on days 6–8 and 4, respectively. In these experiments, the qualitative analysis

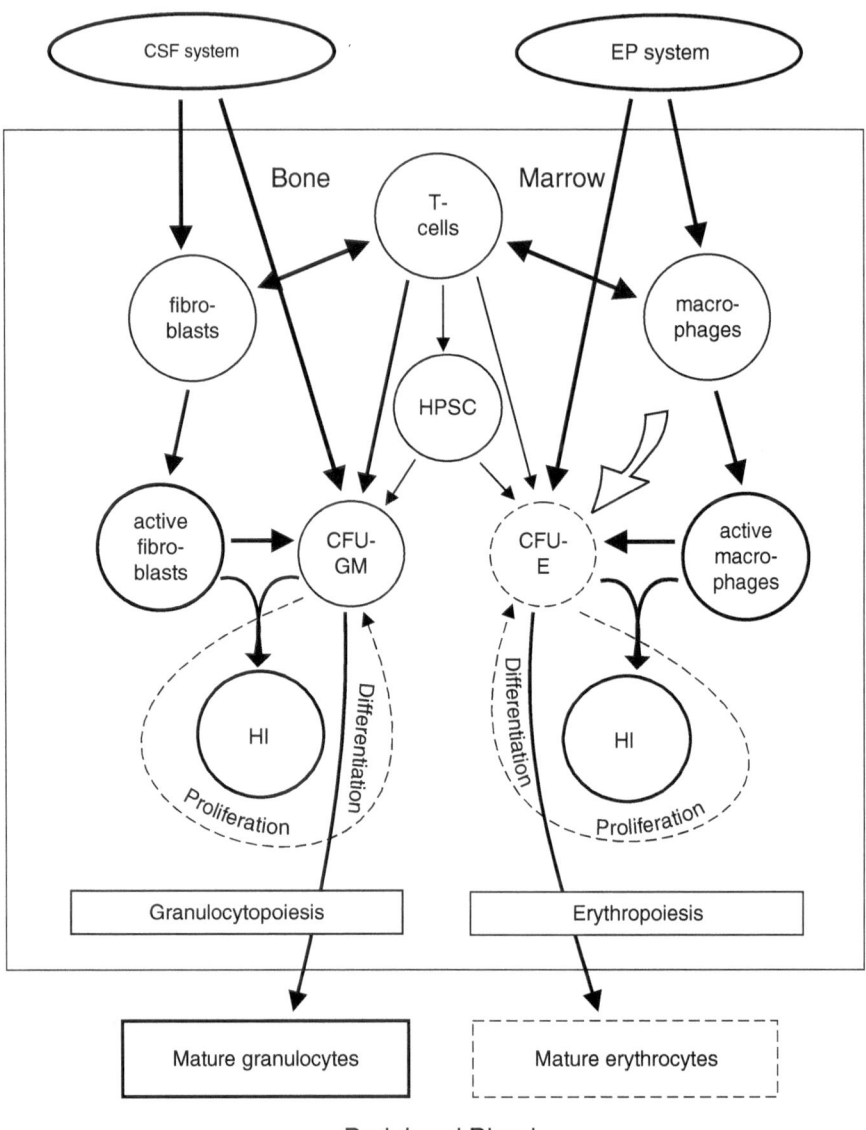

Fig. 6.2 Control of hematopoiesis during severe hypoxia provoking encephalopathia. Absence of any significant changes is marked with fine continuous lines, while the *dash* and *thick solid lines* indicate inhibition and activation, correspondingly. The *open arrow* indicates inhibitory effect by the adrenergic systems

of the blood formed elements revealed a marked decrease in the size of erythrocytes in mice treated with propranolol in comparison with similar value in mice subjected to various types of hypoxia but not treated with this adrenergic blocker.

The revealed alterations in the peripheral blood logically reflected the dynamics of medullar erythropoiesis. For example, treatment of hypoxic mice with propranolol increased the count of erythrocaryocytes in the bone marrow after double hypoxic hypoxia (observed on experiment days 5, 6, 9), hemic hypoxia caused by 150 mg/kg phenylhydrazine (days 6, 7), and hemoexfusion of 70 % circulation blood volume (days 6, 7) in comparison with the animals whose adrenergic mechanisms had not been corrected.

The cell culture studies of the effects of the adrenergic stimuli on erythropoiesis revealed dependence of the above reactions in the blood systems on the state of the progenitor cells in hematopoietic tissue. For instance, propranolol significantly elevated the count of erythroid precursors in the bone marrow on experiment day 4 after hypoxic hypoxia and on days 3–4 after the blood loss. The study of proliferative activity of the hemopoietic progenitor cells revealed an increase of their division rate in all hypoxia models, although it was significant only in the model of hypoxic hypoxia on experiment day 3. At the same time, no group of mice demonstrated significant changes in the rate of CFU-E differentiation despite down-regulation of production of the erythropoietically active substances by the adherent fraction of the bone marrow observed on experiment day 4 after hypoxic hypoxia or blood loss. In these cases, injection of an antagonist of β-adrenergic receptors produced no effect on the secretory function of HIM non-adherent elements and on serum EPA.

However, the alterations in granulomonocytic hemopoietic lineage induced by β-adrenergic antagonist were mostly redistributive in character: they were manifested by the disturbances in the release of immature neutrophils in the blood, which agree with the data obtained in other pathology model [53]. The limited effects of propranolol were manifested only by insignificant accumulation of the mature neutrophilic granulocytes in the bone marrow in the models of hemolytic and severe hemorrhagic anemia, and by a decrease in the count of the rod neutrophils in the peripheral blood observed in the models of hypoxic hypoxia and hemorrhagic anemia. No hypoxia models with the signs of encephalopathia displayed any marked differences in the counts of other morphologically differentiated granulomonocytic cell elements in the bone marrow and peripheral blood or significant diversities in the count and state of CFU-GM pool. Propranolol did not change CSA levels in the conditioned media of the non-adherent myelocaryocytes and in the blood serum, although it down-regulated CSA production by HIM adherent cells on experiment day 5 in the models of hemic hypoxia caused by 150 mg/kg phenylhydrazine and hemorrhagic anemia induced by hemoexfusion of 70 % circulation blood volume.

On the whole, our experiments showed that hyperactivation of the adrenergic systems in an organism subjected to severe hypoxia exerted a negative influence on erythropoiesis. This 'inverse' effect of a surplus of the catecholamines results from the damage to erythroid precursors mediated via β-adrenergic receptors located on their membranes [47, 53].

Thus, the damage to cerebral structures caused by hypoxia and the related alterations in activity of the adrenergic mechanisms of hemopoietic control pronouncedly disturb the development of adequate adaptive reactions in the blood system, which in its turn aggravates the oxygen supply to the tissues in an organism during hypoxia.

Conclusions

The data accumulated on the work of blood systems under normal and pathological conditions show that under the conditions of balanced hemopoiesis, the neuroendocrine substances have no significant effects on the proliferation and differentiation of hemopoietic cells. In such conditions, the hematopoietic system works mostly in an autonomic mode under the predominant control by the local mechanisms.

Under extreme conditions characterized by overstress of the hemopoietic processes, the most important role in sustaining hemopoiesis at an enhanced level is given to the neuroendocrine control systems. They exert both direct (via the corresponding receptors) and indirect (mediated by T-lymphocytes, macrophages, and the stromal elements) effects on the hematopoietic cells resulting in their concerted work and enhancement of their proliferative and differentiating potencies. A salient role in this control belongs to the mediator influences, which are effected, specifically by the monoaminergic systems, where by the serotoninergic system is mostly related to alterations in the erythroid hemopoietic lineage, while the adrenergic and dopaminergic systems are employed to control the changes in granulocytic hemopoietic lineage.

The stressful stimulation activates an integrated cascade mechanism of the hematopoietic control. The role of 'trigger' inducing the adaptive response of the hematopoietic tissue is given to the central neuroendocrine structures exerting their influence via universal stress-mediating (monoaminergic, vegetative, hypophyseal-adrenal, peptide-opioid) and stress-limiting (GABAergic, peptide-opioid, etc.) systems. At this stage, the major player in mediating the vegetative influences on hematopoiesis is the sympathoadrenal system.

The activation of hypophyseal-adrenal and sympathoadrenal systems results in the development of hyperplasia of hemopoietic tissue in the bone marrow (predominantly due to the stimulation of erythro- and granulomonocytopoiesis) accompanied by the enhancement of cellularity of the peripheral blood. The basic reason of hemopoietic activation is the enhancement of migration of T-lymphocyte regulators into the bone marrow under the effect of glucocorticoids and catecholamines. At present,

© Springer International Publishing Switzerland 2014
A.M. Dygai, V.V. Zhdanov, *Theory of Hematopoiesis Control*,
SpringerBriefs in Cell Biology 5, DOI 10.1007/978-3-319-08584-5

the phenotype and basic properties of hemopoietic control T-cells are being examined in detail. T-lymphocytes augment the functional activity of resident macrophages and the stromal mechanocytes that form HIM, which in many respects is responsible for the proliferation and maturation of the cells from progenitor to mature forms. In addition, the hematopoietic control pathways comprise the direct (receptor-based) and indirect (via T-lymphocytes, macrophages, and the stromal mechanocytes) influences of the monoaminergic system and the hormones of the adrenal cortex and medulla on the hematopoietic cells, resulting in synchronization and enhancement of their proliferative and differentiating potencies. A correlation analysis revealed a certain tropicity of α- and β-adrenergic stimulation to granulo-cyte-macrophage and erythroid hemopoietic mechanisms, respectively. The con-certed activity of the stress-mediating and stress-limiting systems directed to corresponding target cells in the blood systems, shapes the adaptive response of the hematopoietic tissue. On the one hand, the resulting alterations are homogenous and non-specific in character, however, the specificity of the blood system response greatly depends on the nature of the pathogenic factor (Figs. 2.1, 2.2, 2.3, 3.1, 3.2, 4.1, 4.2, 4.3, 4.4, 4.5, 4.6, 5.1, 5.2, 5.3, 6.1, and 6.2).

The HIM elements (macrophages and the stromal mechanocytes) in company with T-lymphocytes determines the proliferative and differentiating status of the hemopoietic progenitor cells via the up-regulation in production of the humoral regulators (cytokines and GAG) and enhancement of cell-cell interactions leading to the accelerated formation of the cell associations (HI). It is important to note that one of the earliest HIM reactions observed during stressful stimulation is activation of IL-1 and IL-3 syntheses. At the same time, the number of horizontal (at the level of blood system) and vertical (involving the higher regulator systems) interrelations greatly increases, which restricts the plasticity of the compensation-adaptation hemopoietic mechanisms under these conditions.

Overall, the considered data underlay the hypothetic diagram of hemopoietic control (Fig. 1).

Of principal importance are the roles of local and distant regulator systems in providing the necessary area of hematopoiesis under the normal conditions viewed here as the optimal life of an organism. We are reasonably sure that under balanced hemopoiesis, the neurocrine substances including the central monoaminergic and vegetative transmitters, the hormones of adrenal cortex, and the opioid peptides, produce no direct influence on the proliferative and differentiating status of the hemopoietic cells indicating the virtual autonomic nature of the hematopoietic sys-tem. Specifically, the changes in functional activity of the neuroendocrine apparatus (adrenal cortex and medulla, as well as, the monoaminergic and opiatergic systems) in animals that were not exposed to the stressful stimulation produce no marked effects on hematopoiesis. Similarly, experimental deficiency of T-lymphocytes in an 'intact' organism, which belong to the major links (messengers) of the distant and local hemopoietic control systems, produce no marked effects on hematopoie-sis. However, the anatomic unit referred to as the 'neuroreticular complex' implying involvement of neural terminals in HIM formation suggests the possibility of cer-tain indirect effects of the higher control centers on 'intact' hematopoiesis. This

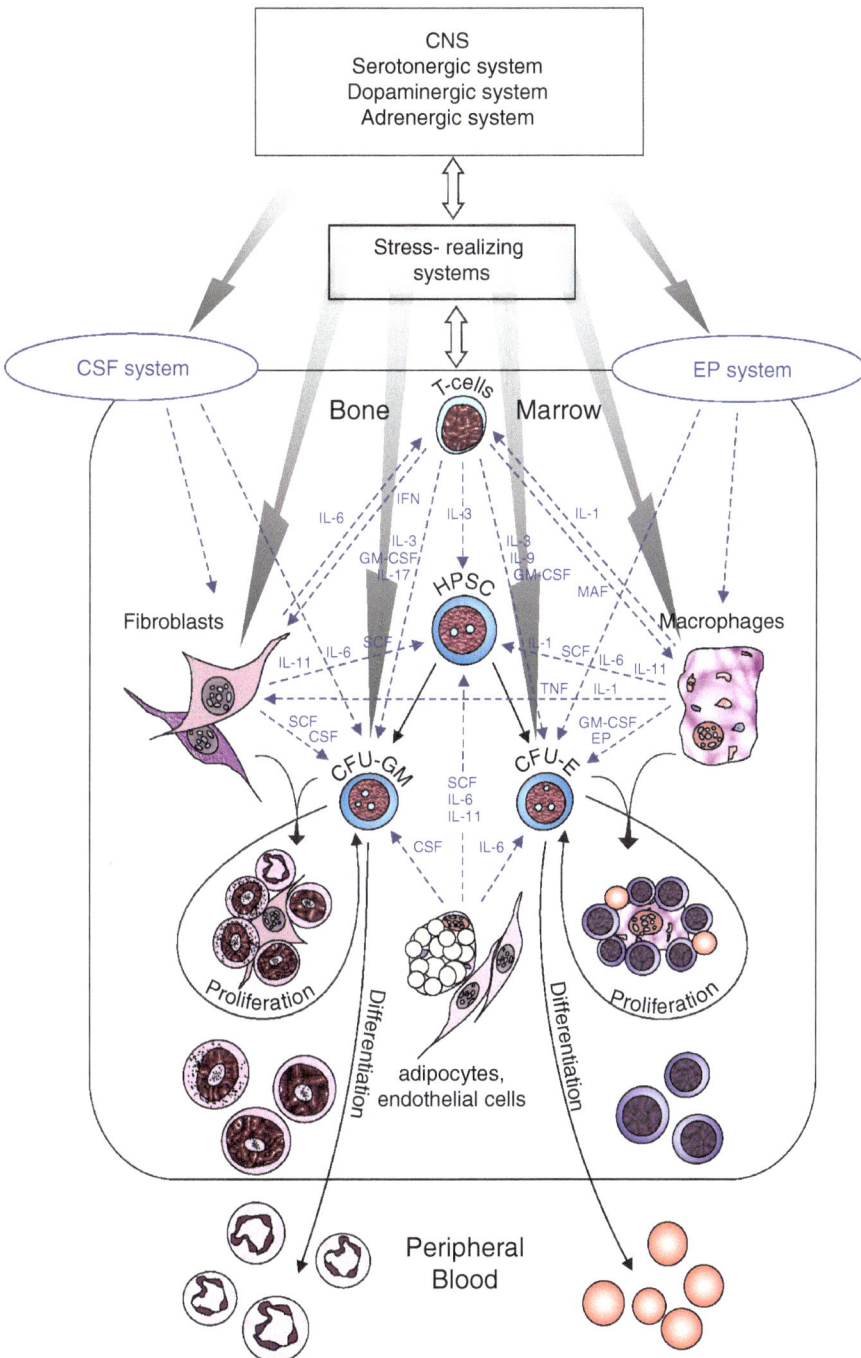

Fig. 1 Control of hematopoiesis in stressed animals

possibility can be realized via the control over metabolism, oxygen consumption, and erythropoietin secretion, as well as, the trophogenic influence on the internal metabolic processes in the cells under a hemopoietic microenvironment, which in turn control the proliferative and differentiating potentials of the hemopoietic elements. Probably, the low levels in production of the hemopoietic humoral regulators by the stromal cells of the bone marrow demonstrates that under normal conditions, they participate in renewal of cell associations via the cell-cell contacts. In this process, the minimum number of horizontal (within bone marrow) and vertical correlation bonds reflects the persistent need of an organism for functionally mature cells of the blood system under the optimal conditions of its vital activity.

Summarizing the short review of the data related to the development of the hemopoietic control theory under stress conditions, it is worth noting that its validity is established by the results of the applied research. For instance, this theory advanced new methods to treat the cytostatic myelosuppressions with neuropharmacological agents, which have been clinically tested [53]. Moreover, a family of novel high efficient hemostimulators has been synthesized on the basis of GAG derivatives [39], the pathogenetic substantiation was developed to use the recombinant forms of cytokines that were successfully employed with the nanotechnology methods to synthetize the principally novel class of the drugs [68, 70, 72], and the hemopoietic control theory was further elaborated to explain the mechanisms of somatization of neuroses [86] and the peculiarities in the development of leucoses [173].

Finally, it can be concluded that hemopoietic tissue is a usable model to examine the regularities in the growth of regenerating tissues, so the key elements of regulation of its activity under normal (optimal) conditions and during stress can be corner-stones in creating the general biological theory of tissue adaptogenesis.

References

1. Agadzhanyan NA, Elfimov AI (1986) Functions of an organism during hypoxia and hypercapnia [in Russian]. Meditsina, Moscow, p 272
2. Agafonov VI, Dygaĭ AM, Shakhov VP, Gol'dberg ED (1994) The role of the hemopoiesis-inducing microenvironment in the postradiation regeneration of hemopoiesis. Radiats Biol Radioekol 34(1):111–116
3. Adyushkin AI (1983) Changes in balance between CFU-S-produced colony types during multiple injections of glucocorticoids at low doses. Gematol Transfuziol 9:32–34
4. Aksinenko SG (1994) The role of sympathetic nervous system in control of hemopoiesis during cytostatic hemosuppression [in Russian]. Abstract of Cand. Med. Sci. Dissertation, Tomsk, p 19
5. Alekseeva AV, Gurvich AM, Semchenko VV (2003) Postresuscitation encephalopathia: pathogenesis, clinical features, prevention, and treatment [in Russian]. Omsk, p 152
6. Almazov VA, Afanas'ev BV, Zaritskii AY, Shishkov AL (1981) Leucopenia [in Russian]. Meditsina, Leningrad, p 240
7. Balitskii KP, Shmal'ko YP (1987) Stress and dissemination of malignant tumors [in Russian]. Naukova Dumka, Kiev, p 24

8. Severin ES (ed) (2005) Textbook on biochemistry [in Russian]. GEOTAR-Media, Moscow, p 784

9. Blokhin NN, Perevodchikova NI (1984) Chemotherapy of tumor diseases [in Russian]. Meditsina, Moscow, p 303

10. Breslav IS, Ivanov AS (1990) Respiration and exercise performance of humans under mountain conditions [in Russian]. Alma-Ata, p 184

11. Brodskiĭ VI, Gusatinskiĭ VN, Kogan AB, Nechaeva NV (1974) Variations in the intensity of H3-leucine incorporation into proteins during slow-wave and paradoxical phases of natural sleep in the cat associative cortex. Dokl Akad Nauk SSSR 215:748–750

12. Bulkina ZP (1991) Antitumor drugs [in Russian]. Naukova Dumka, Kiev, p 304

13. Bures J, Buresova O, Huston JP (1991) Techniques and basic experiments for the study of brain and behavior [Russian translation]. Batuev AS (ed). Vysshaya Shkola, Moscow, p 398

14. Van Leer E, Stikney K (1967) Hypoxia [Russian translation]. Meditsina, Moscow, p 368

15. Vladimirskaya EB, Maschan AA, Rumyantsev AG (1997) Apoptosis and its role in the development of tumor expansion. Gematol Transfuziol 42(5):4–9

16. Vorgalik VG (1953) The studies of Russian scientists on nervous control of blood system [in Russian]. Gorkii, p 64

17. Gavrilov OK, Fainshtein FE, Turbina NS (1987) Suppressions of hematopoiesis [in Russian]. Meditsina, Moscow, p 256

18. Garin AM, Khlebnov AV (1995) Reference book on practical tumor chemotherapy [in Russian]. Moscow, p 304

19. Geĭl RP, Butturini A (1994) Stem cells, clonality, and leukemia. Gematol Transfuziol 39(6):3–6

20. Abdulkadyrov KM (ed) (2004) Hematology: modern reference book [in Russian]. Eksmo/St. Petersburg, Moscow/Sova, p 928

21. Gershanovich ML (1982) Complications during chemo- and hormonotherapy of malignant tumors [in Russian]. Meditsina, Moscow, p 224

22. Goldberg VE, Dygai AM, Novitskii VV (1992) Pulmonary cancer and blood system [in Russian]. TGU, Tomsk, p 236

23. Gol'dberg DI (1952) Essays on hematology (Hemopoiesis and Nervous System) [in Russian]. Tomsk, p 232

24. Gol'dberg DI, Gol'dberg ED (1973) Atlas of bone marrow microphotos during acute radiation disease and action of cytostatic drugs [in Russian]. Meditsina, Moscow, p 143

25. Gol'dberg DI, Zapuskalov VI (1957) The mechanisms of acute leukocyte reaction [in Russian]. Tomsk, p 150

26. Gol'dberg ED (1989) Reference book on hematology with microphoto atlas [in Russian]. TGU, Tomsk, p 486

27. Gol'dberg ED, Dygai AM, Bogdashin IV et al (1987) Phenotypic and functional characteristic of individual subpopulations of T-Lymphocyte regulators under Stress. Actual problems of pharmacology and search for Novel Therapeutic Drugs [in Russian], vol 3. Tomsk, pp 99–101

28. Gol'dberg ED, Dygaĭ AM, Zaritskiĭ AY et al (1988) The role of the stromal microenvironment in regulating bone marrow hemopoiesis under stress. Byull Eksp Biol Med 105(3):270–272

29. Gol'dberg ED, Bel'skiĭ YP, Danilets MG et al (1999) Adaptive potential of granulocytic stem cells in the bone marrow from preleukemic AKR mice. Byull Eksp Biol Med 127(2):151–154

30. Gol'dberg ED, Bel'skiĭ YP, Danilets MG et al (1999) Mechanisms of preleukemic hypoplasia of bone marrow erythroid stem cells in mice AKR/JY. Byull Eksp Biol Med 127(6):633–635

31. Gol'dberg ED, Bel'skiĭ YP, Danilets MG et al (1998) Structure-functional organization of the bone marrow in dynamics of aging of AKR/J mice. Byull Eksp Biol Med 125(3):266–268

32. Gol'dberg ED, Dygai AM (1985) The role of T-lymphocytes in control of proliferation and differentiation of CFU-S, CFU-E, BFU-E. Stem cells and tumor expansion [in Russian]. Naukova Dumka, Kiev, pp 221–225

33. Gol'dberg ED, Dygaĭ AM, Bogdashin IV et al (1991) Role of humoral factors in the regulation of hemopoiesis in stress. Byull Eksp Biol Med 112(7):15–18

34. Gol'dberg ED, Dygai AM, Zhdanov VV (2001) Dynamic theory of hematopoietic control and the role of cytokines in the control of hemopoiesis. Med Immunol 3(4):487–498

35. Gol'dberg ED, Dygai AM, Zhdanov VV (2002) The mechanisms of dysregulation of blood system during pathology. In: Kryzhanovsky GN (ed) Dysregulation pathology: guide book for physicians and biologists [in Russian]. Meditsina, Moscow, pp 386–394

36. Gol'dberg ED, Dygaĭ AM, Zhdanov VV (1998) Mechanisms of hemopoiesis cytostatic damage and regeneration. Vestn Ross Akad Med Nauk 10:6–10

37. Gol'dberg ED, Dygai AM, Zhdanov VV (1999) The role of hemopoietin-inducing microenvironment in hemopoietic control during cytostatic myelosuppressions [in Russian]. STT, Tomsk, p 128

38. Gol'dberg ED, Dygai AM, Zhdanov VV (2005) Modern views on the problem of stem cells and potentialities of their use in medicine. Kletochn Tekhnol Biol Med 4:184–189

39. Gol'dberg ED, Dygai AM, Zhdanov VV et al (2007) Pharmacologic regulation of blood system during experimental neurotic influences [in Russian]. TGU, Tomsk, p 156

40. Gol'dberg ED, Dygaĭ AM, Zhdanov VV, Khlusov IA (1999) Dynamic theory of hemopoiesis. Byull Eksp Biol Med 127(5):484–494

41. Gol'dberg ED, Dygaĭ AM, Zaritskiĭ AY et al (1988) The role of the thymus in regulating the stromal cells responsible for the transfer of the hemopoiesis-inducing microenvironment in stress. Byull Eksp Biol Med 106(12):710–712

42. Gol'dberg ED, Dygaĭ AM, Zakharov YM et al (1991) The specificity of the mechanisms regulating hematopoiesis under different extreme exposures. Patol Fiziol Eksp Ter 3:7–10

43. Gol'dberg ED, Dygai AM, Zyuz'kov GN et al (2002) Mechanisms of changes in the erythroid hemopoietic stem during hypoxias of different severity. Byull Eksp Biol Med 134(8): 142–145

44. Gol'dberg ED, Dygai AM, Karpova GV (1983) The role of lymphocytes in hemopoietic control [in Russian]. TGU, Tomsk, p 160

45. Gol'dberg ED, Dygaĭ AM, Klimenko NA et al (1993) The effect of mast cells on the T-lymphocyte mechanisms of hemopoiesis regulation in inflammation. Byull Eksp Biol Med 115(6):602–604

46. Gol'dberg ED, Dygaĭ AM, Klimenko NA et al (1995) Reaction of erythron and its mechanisms in inflammation. Byull Eksp Biol Med 120(10):382–384

47. Gol'dberg ED, Dygai AM, Provalova NV et al (2004) The role of nervous system in hemopoietic control [in Russian]. TGU, Tomsk, p 146

48. Gol'dberg ED, Dygai AM, Skurikhin EG et al (2000) Adrenergic and cholinergic mechanisms of hemopoiesis regulation during experimental neuroses. Byull Eksp Biol Med 129(4):381–385

49. Skurikhin EG, Pershina OV, Stavrova LA et al (2005) Neurosis-associated changes in the granulocytic hemopoietic stem in mice with different learning capacity. Byull Eksp Biol Med 140(8):136–141

50. Gol'dberg ED, Dygai AM, Suslov NI (1997) Novel drugs based on the products of antler maral breeding [in Russian]. Medical Market 3:5–7

51. Gol'dberg ED, Dygaĭ AM, Udut VV et al (1996) Regularities in structural organization of survival systems in norm and during development of pathological processes [in Russian]. TGU, Tomsk, p 284

52. Gol'dberg ED, Dygaĭ AM, Khlusov IA et al (1993) The production by bone marrow cells of humoral factors in extreme exposures of different origins. Byull Eksp Biol Med 116(9): 244–246

53. Gol'dberg ED, Dygai AM, Khlusov IA (1997) The role of autonomic nervous system in hemopoietic control [in Russian]. TGU, Tomsk, p 219

54. Goldberg ED, Dygai AM, Shakhov VP et al (1987) Structure-functional organization and adaptive mechanisms in hemopoietic system. Bioenergetic and structural aspects of homeostasis in isolated systems and in organism [in Russian]. Krasnoyarsk, pp 75–89

55. Gol'dberg ED, Dygaĭ AM, Shakhov VP (1988) The role of macrophages in the development of the phenomenon of the stimulation of bone marrow hematopoiesis in stress. Patol Fiziol Eksp Ter 5:32–34

56. Gol'dberg ED, Dygai AM, Shakhov VP (1992) Tissue culture methods in hematology [in Russian]. TGU, Tomsk, p 272
57. Gol'dberg ED, Dygai AM, Sherstoboev EY (2000) The mechanisms of local hemopoietic control [in Russian]. STT, Tomsk, p 147
58. Gol'dberg ED, Novitskii VV (1986) Anthracycline-like antitumor antibiotics and blood system [in Russian]. TGU, Tomsk, p 236
59. Gorizontov PD (1981) Blood system as the basis of bodily resistance and adaptation. Patol Fiziol Eksp Ter 2:55–63
60. Gorizontov PD, Белоусова ОИ, Fedotova MI (1983) Stress and blood system [in Russian]. Meditsina, Moscow, p 240
61. Gorizontov PD, Fedotova MI, Belousova OI et al (1980) Effect of exposure to stress on the role of T- and B-lymphocytes in the response of the hematopoietic system. Byull Eksp Biol Med 89(4):416
62. Gubina NA, Morshchakova EF (1974) Molecular aspects of erythropoietic control [in Russian]. Pavlov AD (ed). Ryazan', pp 119–125
63. Gur'yantseva LA, Pozhen'ko NS, Khrichkova TY (2000) Novel drugs as stimulators of granulomonocytopoiesis. Byull Sib Otdel Ross Akad Med Nauk 2:53–58
64. Devoino LV, Idova GV, Al'perina EL et al (2005) Cerebral neurotransmitter systems in modulation of immune response (dopamine, serotonin, GABA). Neiroimmunologiya 3(1):11–18
65. Devoino LV, Il'yuchenok RY (1993) Neurotransmitter systems in psychic immunomodulation: dopamine, serotonin, GABA, and neuropeptides [in Russian]. TsERIS, Novosibirsk, p 240
66. Demin NN, Kogan AB, Moiseeva NI (1978) Neurophysiology and neurochemistry of sleep [in Russian]. Nauka, Leningrad, p 192
67. Dygaĭ AM, Gol'dberg ED, Bogdashin IV et al (1989) Phenotypic and functional characteristics of the subpopulations of regulatory T-lymphocytes participating in the stimulation of hemopoiesis during stress. Byull Eksp Biol Med 107(5):590–593
68. Dygaĭ AM, Artamonov AV, Bekarev AA et al (2011) Nanotechnologies in pharmacology [in Russian]. RAMS Publishing House, Moscow, p 136 p
69. Dygaĭ AM, Buznik DV, Shakhov VP, Gol'dberg ED (1992) The structure-functional organization of the bone marrow after lethal irradiation and the transplantation of syngeneic hematopoietic cells. Radiobiologiya 32(4):575–579
70. Dygai AM, Zhdanov VV (2010) Granulocyte colony-stimulating factor: pharmacological features [in Russian]. RAMS Publishing House, Moscow, p 138
71. Dygai AM, Zhdanov VV, Bogdashin IV, Gol'dberg ED (1992) The role of hemopoietin-inducing microenvironment in the mechanisms of hemopoietic regeneration after cytostatic influence. Biol Nauki 9:109–116
72. Dygaĭ AM, Zhdanov VV, Masycheva VI et al (1999) The blood-simulating properties of a recombinant colony-stimulating factor and glycyram during cytostatic myelosuppression. Eksp Klin Farmakol 62(1):34–37
73. Dygaĭ AM, Zhdanov VV, Minakova MY et al (1997) The role of proliferation and differentiation of the hematopoietic cell precursors during regeneration of hematopoiesis in cytostatic myelosuppression. Byull Eksp Biol Med 124(12):616–620
74. Dygaĭ AM, Zhdanov VV, Minakova MY, Gol'dberg ED (1997) Involvement of humoral factors in the regulation of hematopoiesis in cytostatic myelosuppressions. Byull Eksp Biol Med 124(8):161–165
75. Dygaĭ AM, Zhdanov VV, Khlusov IA et al (1995) Regulating effect of the hematopoiesis-inducing microenvironment on hematopoietic processes as affected by cytostatic drugs. Gematol Transfuziol 40(5):11–15
76. Dygaĭ AM, Ivasenko IN, Ledovskaya SM et al (1988) The role of thymus and hemopoietin-inducing microenvironment in hemopoiesis control under stress. Mechanisms of pathologic reactions [in Russian]. Tomsk, pp 8–11
77. Dygaĭ AM, Kirienkova EV, Mikhlenko AV et al (1986) Role of the thymus in regulating bone marrow hematopoiesis in the stress reaction. Byull Eksp Biol Med 101(4):397–399
78. Dygaĭ AM, Klimenko NA (1992) Inflammation and hemopoiesis [in Russian]. TGU, Tomsk, p 276

79. Dygaĭ AM, Klimenko NA, Abramova EV et al (1991) Blood system responses in inflammation and mechanisms of their development. Patol Fiziol Eksp Ter 6:28–31
80. Dygaĭ AM, Kolokol'tsova TD, Kostina NE et al (2000) Experimental study of hemostimulating properties of the tablet form of recombinant human erythropoietin. Eksp Klin Farmakol 63(5):37–40
81. Dygaĭ AM, Mikhlenko AV, Shakhov VP (1988) The role of T-lymphocytes in regulating the processes of proliferation of the cellular elements in erythro- and granulocytopoiesis in stress. Patol Fiziol Eksp Ter 2:48–51
82. Dygai AM, Skurikhin EG, Pershina OV (2009) Effect of granulocytic colony-stimulating factor on cytostatic-suppressed granulocytopoiesis under conditions of exhausted catecholamine depot. Byull Eksp Biol Med 147(5):540–543
83. Dygai AM, Skurikhin EG, Pershina OV et al (2010) Role of hemopoietic precursors of various classes in the effect of granulocyte colony-stimulating factor on hemopoiesis during cytostatic-induced myelosuppression. Byull Eksp Biol Med 148(4):400–404
84. Dygai AM, Skurikhin EG, Pershina OV et al (2008) Role of central adrenergic structures in the regulation of granulocytopoiesis during cytostatic treatment. Byull Eksp Biol Med 145(4): 383–388
85. Dygai AM, Skurikhin EG, Provalova NV, Suslov NI (2002) Local regulation of proliferation and differentiation of hemopoietic precursors during experimental neurosis. Byull Eksp Biol Med 133(1):17–21
86. Dygai AM, Skurikhin EG, Suslov NI et al (1998) Reactions of granulocytic hematopoietic stem cells during experimental neurosis-inducing situations. Byull Eksp Biol Med 126(12): 628–631
87. Dygai AM, Suslov NI, Skurikhin EG, Churin AA (1997) Reactions of the erythropoietic progenitor cells in various types of neurotic actions. Byull Eksp Biol Med 123(2):158–161
88. Dygai AM, Suslov NI, Skurikhin EG et al (1998) The modulating effects of preparations of Baikal skullcap (Scutellaria baicalensis) on erythron reactions under conditions of neurotic exposures. Eksp Klin Farmakol 61(1):37–39
89. Dygai AM, Udut EV, Zhdanov VV et al (2001) Myelotoxicity of a plant cytostatic preparation etoposide. Eksp Klin Farmakol 64(5):31–33
90. Dygaĭ AM, Shakhov VP (1989) The role of cell-cell interactions in hemopoietic control [in Russian]. TGU, Tomsk, p 224
91. Dygaĭ AM, Shakhov VP, Kirienkova EV et al (1990) The role of glucocorticoids in the development of the phenomenon of bone marrow hematopoiesis stimulation in stress. Biol Nauki 12:71–76
92. Dygaĭ AM, Sherstoboev EY, Gol'dberg ED (1998) The role of SC-1(+)- and Thy-1(+)-cells in the regulation of cytokine production by cells of the bone marrow regenerating after cytostatic action. Byull Eksp Biol Med 125(4):374–377
93. Evtushenko OM, Zhdanov VV (1992) The effect of adriamycin on cytotoxic activity of the cells in mononuclear phagocyte system. Actual problems of pharmacology and search for novel therapeutic preparations [in Russian]. Tomsk, pp 16–19
94. Zakenfel'd GK (1985) The mechanism of immunomodulating effect of zymozan. Unspecific stimulators in tumor immunotherapy [in Russian]. Riga, pp 80–103
95. Zakharov YM (1998) Lections on blood system physiology. Meditsinskii Vestnik [in Russian] 19:152
96. Zakharov YM (2004) The nervous system role in inhibition of hemopoiesis. Ross Fiziol Zh Im I M Sechenova 90(8):987–1000
97. Zakharov YM, Mel'nikov IY (1984) The erythroblastic island–functional-anatomic unit of erythropoiesis. Gematol Transfuziol 29(10):51–56
98. Zakharov YM, Rassokhin AG (2002) Erythroblastic islet [in Russian]. Meditsina, Moscow, p 280
99. Zimin YuI (1979) Immunity and stress. Immunology: pathology of immune system [in Russian], vol 8. Moscow, pp 173–198

100. Zimin YI, Khaitov RM (1975) T-lymphocyte migration into the bone marrow in the initial period of the stress reaction. Byull Eksp Biol Med 80(12):68–70

101. Zyuz'kov GN, Abramova EV, Dygai AM, Gol'dberg ED (2004) Mechanisms of regulation of erythropoiesis during hemolytic anemia. Byull Eksp Biol Med 138(10):378–381

102. Zyuz'kov GN (2006) Hematological mechanisms of adaptation to hypoxia: Abstract of Doct. Med. Sci. Dissertation [in Russian]. Tomsk, p 47

103. Zyuz'kov GN, Abramova EV, Dygai AM, Gol'dberg ED (2005) Reactions of the erythroid hemopoietic stem and their mechanisms during blood loss. Byull Eksp Biol Med 139(1): 32–37

104. Zyuz'kov GN, Gur'yantseva LA, Suslov NI et al (2002) Reactions of hemopoietic granulocytic stem in hypoxia of different severity. Byull Eksp Biol Med 134(10):379–382

105. Zyuz'kov GN, Dygai AM, Gol'dberg ED (2005) Humoral mechanisms of regulation of erythropoiesis during hypoxia. Byull Eksp Biol Med 139(2):133–137

106. Idova GV (1994) The cellular mechanisms of immune modulating effect of neurotransmitter systems. The role of bone marrow. Byull Sib Branch RAMS 4:52–56

107. Idova GV, Cheido MA, Zhukova EN et al (2001) Effects of type 1A serotonin receptor agonist 8-OH-DPAT on immune response. Byull Eksp Biol Med 132(10):432–433

108. Isabaeva VA (1975) Physiology of blood clotting during natural (mountain) adaptation: Abstract of Cand. Med. Sci. Dissertation [in Russian]. Frunze, p 28

109. Kaznacheev VP (1974) Modern problems of human adaptation. Adaptation and the Problems of General Pathology [in Russian], vol 2. Novosibirsk, pp 3–9

110. Karpova GV, Fomina TI, Timina EA et al (1998) The myelotoxicity of vepesid. Eksp Klin Farmakol 61(2):51–53

111. Ketlinskii SA (2002) The role of type 1 and 2 T-helpers in control of cellular and humoral immunity. Immunologiya 2:77–79

112. Kozints GP, Gol'dberg ED (eds) (1982) Kinetic aspects of hemopoiesis [in Russian]. TGU, Tomsk, p 311

113. Kirienkova EV (1986) Roles of corticosteroids and T-lymphocytes in the control of bone marrow hemopoiesis during stress: Abstract of Cand. Med. Sci. Dissertation [in Russian]. Tomsk, p 16

114. Klimenko NA, Dygaĭ AM, Gumilevskii BY et al (1992) Influence of mast cells on the regulatory mechanisms of hemopoietic bone marrow in inflammation. Gematol Transfuziol 4: 16–19

115. Klimenko NA, Dygaĭ AM, Gumilevskii BY et al (1997) Role of mast cells in regulation of erythropoiesis during inflammation. Byull Eksp Biol Med 123(6):626–629

116. Klygul' TA, Krivopalov VA (1966) A device for automatic registration of rat behavior for experimental evaluation of the effect of minor tranquilizers. FarmakolToksikol 2:241–244

117. Koval'zon VM (2003) Explorative activity, stress, and paradoxical sleep. Vestn Biol Psikhiatr 3:3–6

118. Kondratenko NF (1975) Kinetics of the main sections of the hematopoietic system in the process of postradiation regeneration. Byull Eksp Biol Med 80(10):110–112

119. Kryzhanovsky GN (ed) (2002) Dysregulation pathology: guide book for physicians and biologists [in Russian]. Meditsina, Moscow, pp 18–78

120. Kusmartsev SA, Bel'skiĭ YP, Agranovich IM et al (1994) Natural suppressor cells. Usp Sovr Biol 114(6):705–714

121. Kushelevsky VI (1890) The data for medical geography and sanitary description of Fergana region [in Russian]. Novyi Margelan

122. Larionov LF (1972) Side effects of antitumor drugs. Side effects of therapeutic preparations [in Russian] 4:3–28

123. Lebedev VG, Moroz BB, Deshevoĭ YB, Lyrshchikova AV (2004) The role of hematopoietic microenvironment in the mechanism of action of prodigiozan on postradiation recovery of hemopoiesis in long-term bone marrow cultures. Patol Fiziol Eksp Ter 3:7–10

124. Malkin VB, Gipennreiter EB (1977) Acute and chronic hypoxia [in Russian]. Nauka, Moscow, p 315

125. Maianskiĭ AN, Maianskiĭ DN (1989) Essays on neutrophil and macrophage [in Russian]. Nauka, Novosibirsk, p 344

126. Meerson FZ, Pshenichnikova MG (1988) Adaptation to stress exposure and physical loads [in Russian]. Meditsina, Moscow, p 256

127. Melik-Gaikazyan EV (1984) Heterogeneity of Murine Colony-Forming Pool of bone marrow cells under the effect of cytostatic drugs. Actual problems of pharmacology and search of Novel Therapeutic Preparations [in Russian], vol 1. Tomsk, pp 82–86

128. Minakova MYu, Skurikhin EG, Pershina OV (2007) Dopaminergic control of erythropoiesis in modeling myelosuppressions with cyclophosphane and 5-fluorouracil. Byull Eksp Biol Med (Suppl 1):79–86

129. Minakova MYu, Skurikhin EG, Pershina OV, Udut EV (2007) Role of serotoninergic system in the control of erythropoiesis under cytostatic myelosuppressions. Byull Eksp Biol Med (Suppl 1):86–91

130. Miroshnichenko IV (1989) Prethymic development period of T-lymphocytes: properties, maturation, and functions of T-cell progenitors: Abstract of Doct. Biol. Sci. Dissertation [in Russian]. Moscow, p 35

131. Moroz BB, Deshevoĭ YB, Tsybanev OA (1986) Effect of lithium carbonate on the experimental post-radiation recovery of the blood system. Gematol Transfuziol 10:25–29

132. Moroz BB (2002) Postresuscitation disease as dysregulation pathology/dysregulation pathology: guide book for physicians and biologists [in Russian]. Kryzhanovsky GN (ed). Meditsina, Moscow, pp 233–259

133. Nalivaĭko AM (1982) Changes in the rat lymphoid organs in acute hypoxia. Arkh Anat Gistol Embriol 82(6):87–91

134. Natan DG, Ziff KA (1994) Hematopoiesis control. Gematol Transfuziol 39(2):3–10

135. Naumenko OI (1992) Role of bone marrow hemopoietic microenvironment in norm and leucosis. Eksp Onkol 14(1):11–20

136. Novikov NM (1982) Changes in the erythropoiesis-stimulating action of erythrocytic factors in blockade of the mononuclear phagocyte cells. Patol Fiziol Eksp Ter (6):56–58

137. Novitskii VV, Bogdashin IV, Zapuskalova OB et al (1988) Delayed effects of damaging action of antitumor drugs on lymphoid tissue and platelet hemopoietic lineage. Mechanisms of pathologic reactions [in Russian], vol 6. Omsk, pp 57–59

138. Negovsky VA, Gurvich AM, Zolotokrylina ES (1987) Postresuscitation disease [in Russian]. Meditsina, Moscow, p 480

139. Negovsky VA (1991) Neurological aspects of reanimatology. Central nervous system and postresuscitation pathology [in Russian]. Moscow, pp 11–24

140. Ogava M (1990) Hematopoietic stem cells: stochastic differentiation and humoral control of their proliferation. Gematol Transfuziol 35(2):24–30

141. Pavlov AD, Morshchakova EF (1987) Control of erythropoiesis: physiological and clinical aspects [in Russian]. Meditsina, Moscow, p 272

142. Novitskii VV, Gol'dberg ED, Urazova OI (2009) Pathophysiology [in Russian], vol 1. GEOTAR-Media, Moscow, p 848

143. Perevodchikova NI (1993) Antitumor chemotherapy [in Russian]. Meditsina, Moscow, p 223

144. Pershina OV, Skurikhin EG, Stavrova LA et al (2004) Specific features of the erythroid hemopoietic stem in CBA/CaLac mice with neuroses demonstrating good and poor learning capacities. Byull Eksp Biol Med 138(11):499–505

145. Petrov RV, Khaitov RM, Man'ko VM, Mikhailova AA (1981) Control and regulation of immune response [in Russian]. Meditsina, Moscow, p 312

146. Platonova GV, Sof'yanova ZP (1975) Role of carbohydrate component in antitumor features of glycosides. Chemotherapy of tumors in USSR [in Russian] (20):96–100

147. Polenov SA (1986) Hypoxia. Physiology of circulation. Control of circulation [in Russian]. Nauka, Leningrad, pp 384–397

148. Perevodchikova NI (ed) (1996) Antitumor therapy [in Russian]. Moscow, p 223

149. Protsenko LD, Bulkina ZP (1985) Chemistry and pharmacology of synthetic antitumor drugs [in Russian]. Naukova Dumka, Kiev, p 268

150. Romashko OO, Moroz BB, Bezin GI (1979) Stimulating and inhibiting action of hydrocortisone on hematopoietic progenitor cells. Probl Gematol Pereliv Krovi 24(9):48–55

151. Rugal' VI, Blinova TS, Ponomarenko VM, Abdulkadyrov KM (1991) Ultrastructural organization of the hematopoietic microenvironment of human bone marrow. Gematol Transfuziol 36(3):11–15

152. Vorob'ev AI (2002) Textbook on hematology [in Russian], vol 1. Newdiamed, Moscow, p 280

153. Perevodchikova NI (2011) Textbook on chemotherapy of tumor diseases [in Russian]. Prakticheskaya Meditsina, Moscow, p 512

154. Sarkisov DS, Aruin LI (1987) Structural basis of adaptation and compensation for the defective functions [in Russian]. Meditsina, Moscow, pp 20–36

155. Selye H (1960) Studies of the adaptation syndrome [Russian translation]. Medgiz, Moscow, p 254

156. Selye H (1972) At a level of the whole organism [Russian translation]. Meditsina, Moscow, p 121

157. Serov VV, Shekhter AB (1981) Connective tissue [in Russian]. Meditsina, Moscow, p 312

158. Kozlov VA, Sennikov SV (eds) (2004) Cytokine family: theoretical and clinical aspects [in Russian]. Nauka, Novosibirsk, p 324

159. Sverchkova VS (1985) Hypoxia-hypercapnia and functional potencies of an organism [in Russian]. Nauka, Alma-Ata, p 176

160. Skurikhin EG (2004) Mechanisms of hemopoietic control during experimental neuroses: Abstract of Doct. Med. Sci. Dissertation [in Russian]. Tomsk, p 400

161. Skurikhin EG (1997) Reactions of blood system, behavioral abnormalities, and mechanisms of their development during experimental neurosis: Abstract of Cand. Med. Sci. Dissertation [in Russian]. Tomsk, p 211

162. Skurikhin EG, Dygai AM, Provalova NV et al (2005) Mechanisms of regulation of erythropoiesis during experimental neuroses. Byull Eksp Biol Med 139(5):495–501

163. Skurikhin EG, Minakova MY, Pershina OV et al (2007) Dopaminergic regulation of granulocytopoiesis during cytostatic-induced myelosuppressions. Byull Eksp Biol Med 144(9):253–259

164. Skurikhin EG, Pershina OV, Ermakova NN et al (2010) Erythropoiesis-stimulating properties of an antiserotonin drug under cytostatic treatment conditions. Eksp Klin Farmakol 73(3):21–24

165. Skurikhin EG, Pershina OV, Minakova MY et al (2008) Adrenergic regulation of erythropoiesis during cytostatic-induced myelosuppressions. Byull Eksp Biol Med 146(10):385–390

166. Skurikhin EG, Pershina OV, Minakova MYu (2005) Monoaminergic regulation of the pool of erythropoietic stem cells in active and passive mice in experimental neuroses. Kletochn Tekhnol Biol Med (4):247–253

167. Skurikhin EG, Pershina OV, Minakova MY et al (2007) Role of serotonin in the regulation of granulocytopoiesis during cytostatic-induced myelosuppressions. Byull Eksp Biol Med 143(5):501–507

168. Skurikhin EG, Pershina OV, Provalova NV et al (2005) The mechanisms controlling hematopoietic granulocytic lineage in a conflict situation and during deprivation of paradoxical sleep. Byull Eksp Biol Med (Suppl 1):14–20

169. Skurikhin EG, Pershina OV, Suslov NI et al (2005) Role of Thy 1,2+ cells in the regulation of hemopoiesis during experimental neuroses. Byull Eksp Biol Med 139(6):608–612

170. Skurikhin EG, Provalova NV (2000) The role of vegetative Ganglia in hemopoietic control under experimental neuroses. Problems of experimental and clinical pharmacology (Collected papers of Young Researches) [in Russian]. Tomsk, pp 37–38

171. Skurikhin EG, Suslov NI, Provalova NV et al (1999) The role of central adrenergic structures in hemopoietic control under experimental neuroses. Byull Eksp Biol Med 127(Suppl 1):7–11

172. Skurikhin EG, Khmelevskaya ES, Pershina OV et al (2010) Effects of adrenomimetics and serotonin on pluripotent stromal and hemopoietic precursors in cytostatic myelosuppression. Kletochn Tekhnol Biol Med (3):127–132

173. Stavrova LA, Dygai AM, Zhdanov VV et al (2001) Role of mononuclear phagocyte system in hemopoiesis regulation in AKR/JY mice during preleukemic period. Byull Eksp Biol Med 131(1):52–54

174. Suslov NI, Gur'yanov YuG (2004) Therapeutic products based on pantohematogen: mechanisms of action and peculiarities of employment [in Russian]. Novosibirsk, p 144

175. Tilis AYu, Kydyrmaev BK (1978) Effect of high-altitude adaptation on interaction between erythro- and leucopoiesis. Regulatory mechanisms in blood system [in Russian], Part 1. Krasnoyarsk, pp 157–158

176. Totolyan AA, Freidlin IS (2000) The cells of immune system [in Russian]. Nauka, St. Petersburg, p 231

177. Trentin DD (1982) The hematopoietic microenvironment. Probl Gematol Pereliv Krovi 27(7):52–57

178. Tulebekov BT, Norimov AS (1980) Stem cells and T- and B-lymphocytes in acute hypoxia. Byull Eksp Biol Med 40(8):15–17

179. Udut EV, Zhdanov VV, Gur'yantseva LA et al (2001) Role of hemopoietic growth factors in regeneration of hemopoiesis during etoposide-induced myelosuppression. Byull Eksp Biol Med 131(5):512–516

180. Uzhanskiĭ YG, Novikov NM, Yushkov BG (1977) Effect of erythrocyte breakdown products on stem cells and erythropoietin formation. Byull Eksp Biol Med 84(8):143–145

181. Fridenshtein AY, Luriya EA (1980) Cellular basis of hemopoietic microenvironment [in Russian]. Meditsina, Moscow, p 213

182. Khlusov IA, Dygaí AM, Gol'dberg ED (1997) Adrenergic dependence of hematopoietic precursors proliferation under cytostatic effect. Byull Eksp Biol Med 123(6):638–641

183. Khlusov IA, Raskovalova TY, Kirienkova EV, Dygai AM (1999) Effect of adrenals on the hematopoietic microenvironment of the bone marrow. Byull Eksp Biol Med 128(11): 586–590

184. Cheĭdo MA (1997) The role of dopaminergic mechanism in the realization of immunostimulating effect of substance P and its analog. Byull Eksp Biol Med 123(2):135–137

185. Chekalova YI, Ryabova LV (1981) Interaction between syngeneic hemopoietic stem cells and lymphocytes in leukemic AKR mice. Byull Eksp Biol Med 92(12):707–709

186. Cheredeev AN (1990) Interleukins: functional role as mediators of the immune system. Lab Delo 10:4–11

187. Chernigovsky VN, Shekhter SYu, Yaroshevsky AYa (1967) Control of erythropoiesis [in Russian]. Leningrad, p 101

188. Chernigovsky VN, Yaroshevsky AY (1953) Problems of neural control of blood system [in Russian]. Medgiz, Moscow, p 222

189. Chertkov IL, Deryugina EI, Levir RD, Abrakham NG (1991) Stem hemopoietic cell: differentiating and proliferative potential. Usp Sovr Biol 111(6):905–922

190. Shakhov VP (1988) On the control mechanism of hemopoietic islet function under stressinduced adaptive rearrangement of the bone marrow. Stem hemopoietic cell in norm and pathology [in Russian]. Tomsk, pp 26–28

191. Shakhov VP (1990) Role of hemopoietin-inducing microenvironment in control of proliferation and differentiation of myelopoiesis progenitor cells during stress: Abstract of Doct. Med. Sci. Dissertation [in Russian]. Tomsk, p 27

192. Shakhov VP, Dygaí AM, Mikhlenko AV et al (1986) Role of the thymus gland in the regulation of the processes of proliferation and differentiation of various types of precursor cells of myelopoiesis in stress. Patol Fiziol Eksp Ter 5:24–27

193. Epshtein OI, Shtark MB, Dygai AM et al (2005) Pharmacology of ultra-Low doses of antibodies against endogenous functional regulators [in Russian]. RAMS Publishing House, Moscow, p 225

194. Epshtein OI, Dygai AM, Zhdanov VV et al (2007) A comparative study of stimulation of erythropoiesis during renal anemia with the preparation of antibodies against erythropoietin in ultralow doses and Recormon. Byull Eksp Biol Med 143(6):641–644

195. Yudin AM (1993) Pants and antlers: horns as crude drugs [in Russian]. Nauka, Novosibirsk, p 120

196. Yushkov BG, Klimin VG, Severin MV (1999) Blood system and stressful stimulation of an organism [in Russian]. Yekaterinburg, p 198

197. Yushkov BG, Klimin VG, Kuz'min AI (2004) Blood vessels in bone marrow and hemopoietic control [in Russian]. Ural Division of RAS, Yekaterinburg, p 150

198. Yastrebov AP, Yushkov BG, Bol'shakov VN (1988) Control of hemopoiesis in organism exposed to extreme stimuli [in Russian]. Sverdlovsk, p 152

199. Abbas AK, Murphy KM, Sher A (1996) Functional diversity of helper T-lymphocytes. Nature 383(6603):787–793

200. Abdul Hamied TA, Turk JL (1987) Enhancement of interleukin-2 release in rats by treatment with bleomycin and adriamycin in vivo. Cancer Immunol Immunother 25(3):245–249

201. Adelman DM, Maltepe E, Simon MC (1999) Multilineage embryonic hematopoiesis requires hypoxic ARNT activity. Genes Dev 13(19):2478–2483

202. Angelin-Duclos C, Domenget C, Kolbus A et al (2005) Thyroid hormone T3 acting through the thyroid hormone alpha receptor is necessary for implementation of erythropoiesis in the neonatal spleen environment in the mouse. Development 132(5):925–934

203. Arai F, Hirao A, Ohmura M et al (2004) Tie2/angiopoietin-1 signaling regulates hematopoietic stem cell quiescence in the bone marrow niche. Cell 118(2):149–161

204. Arai F, Hirao A, Suda T (2005) Regulation of hematopoiesis and its interaction with stem cell niches. Int J Hematol 82(5):371–376

205. Arnold JT, Barber L, Bertoncello I, Williams NT (1995) Modified thrombopoietic response to 5-FU in mice following transplantation of Lin-Sca-1+ bone marrow cells. Exp Hematol 23(2):161–167

206. Athlin L, Domellof L, Norberg B (1989) Effect of therapeutic concentrations of anthracyclines on monocyte phagocytosis of yeast cells. Eur J Clin Pharmacol 36(2):155–159

207. Belkacemi Y, Bouchet S, Frick J et al (2003) Monitoring of residual hematopoiesis after total body irradiation in humans as a model for accidental x-ray exposure: dose-effect and failure of ex vivo expansion of residual stem cells in view of autografting. Int J Radiat Oncol Biol Phys 57(2):500–507

208. Blau CA, Neff T, Papayannopoulou T (1996) The hematological effects of folate analogs: implications for using the dihydrofolate reductase gene for in vivo selection. Hum Gene Ther 7(17):2069–2078

209. Blazsek I, Liu XH, Anjo A (1995) The hematon, a morphogenetic functional complex in mammalian bone marrow, involves erythroblastic islands and granulocytic cobblestones. Exp Hematol 23(4):309–319

210. Bodey B, Bodey B Jr, Siegel SE, Kaiser HE (2000) The role of the reticulo-epithelial (RE) cell network in the immuno-neuroendocrine regulation of intrathymic lymphopoiesis. Anticancer Res 20(3A):1871–1888

211. Bodey B, Siegel SE, Kaiser HE (2002) Restoration of the thymic cellular microenvironment following autologous bone marrow transplantation. In Vivo 16(2):127–140

212. Bogliolo G, Muzzulini C, Lerza R, Pannacciulli I (1986) Activity of doxorubicin linked to poly-L-aspartic acid on normal murine hematopoietic progenitor cells. Cancer Treat Rep 70(11):1275–1281

213. Borojevic R, Roela RA, Rodarte RS et al (2004) Bone marrow stroma in childhood myelodysplastic syndrome: composition, ability to sustain hematopoiesis in vitro, and altered gene expression. Leuk Res 28(8):831–844

214. Brandan N, Aguirre M, Carmuega R et al (1997) Proliferative and maturative behaviour patterns on murine bone marrow and spleen erythropoiesis along hypoxia. Acta Physiol Pharmacol Ther Latinoam 47(2):125–135

215. Broome CS, Miyan JA (2000) Neuropeptide control of bone marrow neutrophil production. A key axis for neuroimmunomodulation. Ann N Y Acad Sci 917:424–434

216. Burek B, Hrsak I (1995) In vitro modulation of preleukemic AKR mouse macrophage function by bacterial immunomodulators. Immunol Lett 45(3):185–188

217. Bussolino F, Bocchietto E, Silvagno F et al (1994) Actions of molecules which regulate hemopoiesis on endothelial cells: memoirs of common ancestors? Pathol Res Pract 190(9–10):834–839

218. Caldwell J, Emerson SG (1994) IL-1 alpha and TNF alpha act synergistically to stimulate production of myeloid colony-stimulating factors by cultured human bone marrow stromal cells and cloned stromal cell strains. J Cell Physiol 159(2):221–228

219. Campbell AD, Long MW, Wicha MS (1990) Developmental regulation of granulocytic cell binding to hemonectin. Blood 76(9):1758–1764

220. Cecchini MG, Hofstetter W, Halasy J et al (1997) Role of CSF-1 in bone and bone marrow development. Mol Reprod Dev 46(1):75–83

221. Chopra IJ (1981) Triiodothyronines in health and disease. Monogr Endocrinol 18(1–14):58–145

222. Cipolleschi MG, D'Ippolito G, Bernabei PA et al (1997) Severe hypoxia enhances the formation of erythroid bursts from human cord blood cells and the maintenance of BFU-E in vitro. Exp Hematol 25(11):1187–1194

223. Cohen JJ (1972) Thymus-derived lymphocytes sequestered in the bone marrow of hydrocortisone-treated mice. J Immunol 108(3):841–844

224. Colinas RJ, Burkart PT, Lawrence DA (1994) In vitro effects of hydroquinone, benzoquinone, and doxorubicin on mouse and human bone marrow cells at physiological oxygen partial pressure. Toxicol Appl Pharmacol 129(1):95–102

225. Consolo F, Princi P (1960) Experimental research on the action of corticoids and of ACTH on normal bone marrow activity. Boll Soc Ital Biol Sper 36:531–534

226. Coviello AD, Kaplan B, Lakshman KM et al (2008) Effects of graded doses of testosterone on erythropoiesis in healthy young and older men. J Clin Endocrinol Metab 93(3):914–919

227. Crocker PR, Gordon S (1985) Isolation and characterization of resident stromal macrophages and hematopoietic cell clusters from mouse bone marrow. J Exp Med 162(3):993–1014

228. Dal-Zotto S, Marti O, Armario A (2003) Glucocorticoids are involved in the long-term effects of a single immobilization stress on the hypothalamic-pituitary-adrenal axis. Psychoneuroendocrinology 28(8):992–1009

229. Dexter TM (1989) Haemopoietic growth factors. Br Med Bull 45(2):337–349

230. Doiron AL, Kirkpatrick AP, Rinker KD (2004) TGF-beta and TNF-a affect cell surface proteoglycan and sialic acid expression on vascular endothelial cells. Biomed Sci Instrum 40:331–336

231. Donahue RE, Yang YC, Clark SC (1990) Human P40 T-cell growth factor (interleukin-9) supports erythroid colony formation. Blood 75(12):2271–2275

232. Dudley ME, Wunderlich JR, Yang JC et al (2002) A phase I study of nonmyeloablative chemotherapy and adoptive transfer of autologous tumor antigen-specific T lymphocytes in patients with metastatic melanoma. J Immunother 25(3):243–251

233. Dygai AM, Khlusov IA, Udut VV et al (1997) Regulating effect of sympathetic-adrenal system on hemopoiesis suppressed by cytostatic drugs. Pathophysiology 4:175–181

234. Egrie JC, Dwyer E, Browne JK et al (2003) Darbepoetin alfa has a longer circulating half-life and greater in vivo potency than recombinant human erythropoietin. Exp Hematol 31(4):290–299

235. Ehrenbourg I, Gorbatchenkov A (1993) Interval hypoxic training of patients with coronary heart disease. Hypoxia Med J 1:14–18

236. Favier R, Spielvogel H, Caceres E et al (1997) Differential effects of ventilatory stimulation by sex hormones and almitrine on hypoxic erythrocytosis. Pflugers Arch 434(1):97–103

237. Fauci AS, Dale DC (1974) The effect of in vivo hydrocortisone on subpopulations of human lymphocytes. J Clin Invest 53(1):240–246

238. Fearon DT, Locksley RM (1996) The instructive role of innate immunity in the acquired immune response. Science 272(5258):50–53

239. Fink GD, Fisher JW (1976) Erythropoietin production after renal denervation or beta-adrenergic blockade. Am J Physiol 230(2):508–513

240. Fisher JW, Crook JJ (1962) Influence of several hormones on erythropoiesis and oxygen consumption in the hypophysectomized rat. Blood 19:557–565

241. Frolov NA, Shebalin AI, Letchamo W (2000) Eurasian perspective on antler nutraceuticals for the newly emerging functional food market (panto project): history, development and current status of the velvet antler industry in Russia. The 1st International symposium on Antler Science and Product Technology. Abstracts. Banff Centre, Banff, p 42

242. Gardner RV, McKinnon E, Poretta C, Leiva L (2003) Hemopoietic function after use of IL-1 with chemotherapy or irradiation. J Immunol 171(3):1202–1206

243. Gervais V, Zerial A, Oschkinat H (1997) NMR investigations of the role of the sugar moiety in glycosylated recombinant human granulocyte-colony-stimulating factor. Eur J Biochem 247(1):386–395

244. Giltay EJ, Gooren LJ (2009) Potential side effects of androgen deprivation treatment in sex offenders. J Am Acad Psychiatry Law 37(1):53–58

245. Gimble JM, Robinson CE, Wu X, Kelly KA (1996) The function of adipocytes in the bone marrow stroma: an update. Bone 19(5):421–428

246. Gimble JM, Zvonic S, Floyd ZE et al (2006) Playing with bone and fat. J Cell Biochem 98(2):251–266

247. Glader BE, Rambach WA, Alt HL (1968) Observations on the effect of testosterone and hydrocortisone on erythropoiesis. Ann N Y Acad Sci 149(1):383–388

248. Gol'dberg ED, Dygai AM, Suslov NI et al (2000) Pantogematogen (PG): a new formula from maral, Siberian red deer blood. The 1-st international symposium on Antler Science and Product Technology. Abstracts. Banff Centre, Banff, p 35

249. Goldberg ED, Dygai AM (1994) Cytokines production by regenerating bone marrow cells after cytostatic action. Pathophysiology 1:3–23

250. Goldberg ED, Dygai AM (1992) Hemopoiesis regulation mechanisms under stress: hematology reviews, vol 4. London, pp 11–67

251. Goldberg ED, Dygai AM, Klimenko NA (1998) Inflammation and the blood system: hematology reviews, vol 7 (Pt. 4). London, pp 1–75

252. Golde DW, Bersch N, Quan SG, Cline MJ (1976) Inhibition of murine granulopoiesis in vitro by dexamethasone. Am J Hematol 1(4):369–373

253. Goldman S, Loebelenz J, McCarthy K et al (1991) Recombinant human interleukin-11 stimulates megakaryocyte maturation and increase in peripheral platelet number in vivo. Blood 78(10):132

254. Gordon AS, Mirand EA, Zanjani ED (1967) Mechanisms of prednisolone action in erythropoiesis. Endocrinology 81(2):363–368

255. Gordon MY (1988) Extracellular matrix of the marrow microenvironment. Br J Haematol 70(1):1–4

256. Gordon MY (1994) Stem cells and the microenvironment in aplastic anaemia. Br J Haematol 86(1):190–192

257. Greco FA, Brereton HD (1977) Effect of lithium carbonate on the neutropenia caused by chemotherapy: a preliminary clinical trial. Oncology 34(4):153–155

258. Greenberger JS, Wroble LM, Sakakeeny MA (1980) Murine leukemia viruses: induction of macrophage production of granulocyte-macrophage colony-stimulating factor in vitro. J Natl Cancer Inst 65(4):841–851

259. Gregoretti MG, Gottardi D, Ghia P et al (1994) Characterization of bone marrow stromal cells from multiple myeloma. Leuk Res 18(9):675–682

260. Grohmann U, Van Snick J, Campanile F et al (2000) IL-9 protects mice from Gram-negative bacterial shock: suppression of TNF-alpha, IL-12, and IFN-gamma, and induction of IL-10. J Immunol 164(8):4197–4203

261. Gu YC, Kortesmaa J, Tryggvason K et al (2003) Laminin isoform-specific promotion of adhesion and migration of human bone marrow progenitor cells. Blood 101(3):877–885

262. Haas R, Schmid H, Hahn U et al (1997) Tandem high-dose therapy with ifosfamide, epirubicin, carboplatin and peripheral blood stem cell support is an effective adjuvant treatment for high-risk primary breast cancer. Eur J Cancer 33(3):372–378

263. Hager ED, Dziambor H, Winkler P et al (2002) Effects of lithium carbonate on hematopoietic cells in patients with persistent neutropenia following chemotherapy or radiotherapy. J Trace Elem Med Biol 16(2):91–97

264. Halvorsen S (1961) Plasma erythropoietin levels following hypothalamic stimulation in the rabbit. Scand J Clin Lab Invest 13:564–575

265. Halvorsen S (1966) The central nervous system in regulation of erythropoiesis. Acta Haematol 35(2):65–79

266. Hardy CL, Minguell JJ (1993) Cellular interactions in hemopoietic progenitor cell homing: a review. Scanning Microsc 7(1):333–341

267. Hartley C, Elliott S, Begley CG et al (2003) Kinetics of hematopoietic recovery after dose-intensive chemo/radiotherapy in mice: optimized erythroid support with darbepoetin alpha. Br J Haematol 122(4):623–636

268. Hasan NM, Parker PJ, Adams GE (1996) Induction and phosphorylation of protein kinase C-alpha and mitogen-activated protein kinase by hypoxia and by radiation in Chinese hamster V79 cells. Radiat Res 145(2):128–133

269. Haylock DN, Nilsson SK (2006) Osteopontin: a bridge between bone and blood. Br J Haematol 134(5):467–474

270. Haylock DN, Nilsson SK (2005) Stem cell regulation by the hematopoietic stem cell niche. Cell Cycle 4(10):1353–1355

271. Hellebostad M, Ostbye KM, Halvorsen S (1992) Leukemia and anemia in AKR/O mice. II Role of the spleen as an erythropoietic organ during leukemia development. APMIS 100(2):181–187

272. Hellebostad M, Sanengen T, Halvorsen S (1990) Variations in erythropoiesis throughout a lifetime. Studies in a high-leukaemic mouse strain, the AKR/O strain, and a non-leukemic strain, the WLO strain. Blood 61(6):358–363

273. Hill AD, Naama HA, Calvano SE, Daly JM (1995) The effect of granulocyte-macrophage colony-stimulating factor on myeloid cells and its clinical applications. J Leukoc Biol 58(6):634–642

274. Ihara T, Tsujikawa T, Hodohara K et al (1996) Severe anemia in a patient with isolated adrenocorticotropin deficiency. Intern Med 35(11):898–901

275. Ivanovic Z, Bartolozzi B, Bernabei PA et al (2000) Incubation of murine bone marrow cells in hypoxia ensures the maintenance of marrow-repopulating ability together with the expansion of committed progenitors. Br J Haematol 108(2):424–429

276. Jackowski S, Rettenmier CW, Rock CO (1990) Prostaglandin E2 inhibition of growth in a colony-stimulating factor 1-dependent macrophage cell line. J Biol Chem 265(12):6611–6616

277. Jacobsen FW, Smeland EB, Jacobsen SE (1993) TNF-α is a potent inhibitor of murine HPP-CFC stimulated by SCF and other hematopoietic growth factors. J Cell Biochem (Suppl 17b):64

278. Janczewska S, Ziolkowska A, Interewicz B et al (2000) Vascularized bone marrow transplanted in orthotopic hind-limb stimulates hematopoietic recovery in total-body-irradiated rats. Transpl Int 13(Suppl 1):S541–546

279. Jelkmann W (1994) Biology of erythropoietin. Clin Investig 72(6 Suppl):S3–10

280. Jelkmann W, Metzen E (1996) Erythropoietin in the control of red cell production. Ann Anat 178(5):391–403

281. Johnson D, Montpetit ML, Stocker PJ, Bennett ES (2004) The sialic acid component of the beta1 subunit modulates voltage-gated sodium channel function. J Biol Chem 279(43):44303–44310

282. Jouvet D, Vimont P, Delorme F, Jouvet M (1964) Study of selective deprivation of the paradoxal sleep phase in the cat. C R Seances Soc Biol Fil 158:756–759

283. Kacena MA, Gundberg CM, Horowitz MC (2006) A reciprocal regulatory interaction between megakaryocytes, bone cells, and hematopoietic stem cells. Bone 39(5):978–984

284. Kanbe E, Hatta Y, Tsuboi I et al (2006) Effects of neopterin on the hematopoietic microenvironment of senescence-accelerated mice (SAM). Biol Pharm Bull 29(1):43–48

285. Kania K, Dragojew S, Jozwiak Z (2003) Morphological and biochemical changes in human fibroblast lines induced by anthracyclines during apoptosis. Cell Mol Biol Lett 8(1):121–126

286. Kazuto Y, Terence D (1990) Ultrastructural morphometric study of efferent nerve terminal on murine bone marrow stromal cells, and the recognition of a novel anatomical unit: the Neuro-Reticular Complex. Am J Anat 187(3):261–277

287. Keller DC, Du XX, Srour EF et al (1993) Interleukin-11 inhibits adipogenesis and stimulates myelopoiesis in human long-term marrow cultures. Blood 82(5):1428–1435

288. Kim SY, Evans LH, Malik FG, Rouse RV (1991) Macrophages are the first thymic cells to express polytropic retrovirus in AKR mouse leukemogenesis. J Virol 65(11):6238–6241

289. Kinik ST, Ozbek N, Yucel M et al (2005) Correlations among serum leptin levels, complete blood count parameters and peripheral CD34(+) cell count in prepubertal obese children. Ann Hematol 84(9):605–608

290. Kobayashi M, Imamura M, Uede T et al (1994) Expression of adhesion molecules on human hematopoietic progenitor cells at different maturational stages. Stem Cells 12(3):316–321

291. Konar DB, Manchanda SK (1970) Role of hypothalamus in the phagocytic activity of the reticulo-endothelial system. Ind J Physiol Pharmacol 14(2):23–24

292. Koury MJ, Bondurant MC (1988) Maintenance by erythropoietin of viability and maturation of murine erythroid precursor cells. J Cell Physiol 137(1):65–74

293. Krantz SB (1991) Erythropoietin. Blood 77(3):419–434

294. Krantz SB, Jacobson LO (1970) Erythropoietin and the regulation of erythropoiesis. University of Chicago Press, Chicago

295. Kriegler AB, Bernardo D, Verschoor SM (1994) Protection of murine bone marrow by dexamethasone during cytotoxic chemotherapy. Blood 83(1):65–71

296. Lacombe C, Da Silva JL, Bruneval P et al (1988) Peritubular cells are the site of erythropoietin synthesis in the murine hypoxic kidney. J Clin Invest 81(2):620–623

297. Laharrague P, Oppert JM, Brousset P et al (2000) High concentration of leptin stimulates myeloid differentiation from human bone marrow CD34+ progenitors: potential involvement in leukocytosis of obese subjects. Int J Obes Relat Metab Disord 24(9):1212–1216

298. Lai YH, Heslan JM, Poppema S et al (1996) Continuous administration of Il-13 to mice induces extramedullary hemopoiesis and monocytosis. J Immunol 156(9):3166–3173

299. Lau AS, Lehman D, Geertsma FR, Yeung MC (1996) Biology and therapeutic uses of myeloid hematopoietic growth factors and interferons. Pediatr Infect Dis J 15(7):563–575

300. Landi S (1997) Psychoactivator 'Pantogematogen'. J Plant Nutr 20(2–3):311–326

301. Leary AG, Ikebuchi K, Hirai Y et al (1988) Synergism between interleukin-6 and interleukin-3 in supporting proliferation of human hematopoietic stem cells: comparison with interleukin-1 alpha. Blood 71(6):1759–1763

302. Levesque JP, Leavesley DI, Niutta S et al (1995) Cytokines increase human hemopoietic cell adhesiveness by activation of very late antigen (VLA)-4 and VLA-5 integrins. J Exp Med 181(5):1805–1815

303. Li C, Jackson RM (2002) Reactive species mechanisms of cellular hypoxia-reoxygenation injury. Am J Physiol Cell Physiol 282(2):C227–C241

304. Li WM, Huang WQ, Huang YH et al (2000) Positive and negative hematopoietic cytokines produced by bone marrow endothelial cells. Cytokine 12(7):1017–1023

305. Lisukov IA, Tsyrlova IG, Kozlov VA (1986) Effect of androgens on the development of leukemia in AKR-strain mice. Eksp Onkol 8(1):71–73, 79

306. Lohrmann HP, Schreml W (1982) Cytotoxic drugs and the granulopoietic system. Springer, Berlin

307. Lothrop CD Jr, Coulson PA, Nolan HL et al (1987) Cyclic hormonogenesis in gray collie dogs: interactions of hematopoietic and endocrine systems. Endocrinology 120(3):1027–1032

308. Lovschall H, Kassem M, Mosekilde L (1997) Apoptosis: molecular aspects. Nord Med 112(8):271–275

309. Luck HJ, Du Bois A, Thomssen C (1997) Paclitaxel and epirubicin as first-line therapy for patients with metastatic breast cancer. Oncology (Williston Park) 11(4 Suppl 3):34–37

310. Maciejewski JP, Selleri C, Sato T et al (1995) Nitric oxide suppression of human hematopoiesis in vitro. Contribution to inhibitory action of interferon-gamma and tumor necrosis factor-alpha. J Clin Invest 96(2):1085–1092

311. Maestroni GJ, Togni M, Covacci V (1997) Norepinephrine protects mice from acute lethal doses of carboplatin. Exp Hematol 25(6):491–494

312. Maestroni GJ, Conti A (1994) Modulation of hematopoiesis via alpha 1-adrenergic receptors on bone marrow cells. Exp Hematol 22(3):313–320

313. Majumdar MK, Thiede MA, Haynesworth SE et al (2000) Human marrow-derived mesenchymal stem cells (MSCs) express hematopoietic cytokines and support long-term hematopoiesis when differentiated toward stromal and osteogenic lineages. J Hematother Stem Cell Res 9(6):841–848

314. Malacrida SA, Teixeira NA, Queiroz ML (1997) Regulation of stress-induced reduced myelopoiesis in rats. Int J Immunopharmacol 19(4):227–233

315. Mantovani A, Sozzani S, Locati M et al (2002) Macrophage polarization: tumor-associated macrophages as a paradigm for polarized M2 mononuclear phagocytes. Trends Immunol 23(11):549–555

316. Maslova LN, Naumenko EV (1997) The role of glucocorticoids in a modification of the hypothalamo-hypophyseal-adrenal cortical function of rats induced by stress exposures in early ontogeny. Ross Fiziol Zh Im I M Sechenova 83(8):80–86

317. Mayani H (1996) Composition and function of the hemopoietic microenvironment in human myeloid leukemia. Leukemia 10(6):1041–1047

318. McNiece IK, Langley KE, Zsebo KM (1991) Recombinant human stem cell factor synergizes with GM-CSF, G-CSF, IL-3 and epo to stimulate human progenitor cells of the myeloid and erythroid lineages. Exp Hematol 19(3):226–231

319. Metcalf D (1960) Adrenal cortical function in high- and low-leukemia strains of mice. Cancer Res 20:1347–1353

320. Metcalf D (1989) Haemopoietic growth factors 1. Lancet 1(8642):825–827

321. Mide SM, Huygens P, Bozzini CE, Fernandez Pol JA (2001) Effects of human recombinant erythropoietin on differentiation and distribution of erythroid progenitor cells on murine medullary and splenic erythropoiesis during hypoxia and post-hypoxia. In Vivo (Greece) 15(2):125–132

322. Minguell JJ, Erices A, Conget P (2001) Mesenchymal stem cells. Exp Biol Med (Maywood) 226(6):507–520

323. Mladenovic J, Adamson JW (1984) Adrenergic modulation of erythropoiesis: in vitro studies of colony-forming cells in normal and polycythaemic man. Br J Haematol 56(2): 323–332

324. Mohle R, Rafii S, Moore MA (1998) The role of endothelium in the regulation of hematopoietic stem cell migration. Stem Cells 16(Suppl 1):159–165

325. Morley A, Stohlman F Jr (1970) Cyclophosphamide-induced cyclical neutropenia. An animal model of a human periodic disease. N Engl J Med 282(12):643–646

326. Mosmann TR, Cherwinski H, Bond MW et al (1986) Two types of murine helper T cell clone. I. Definition according to profiles of lymphokine activities and secreted proteins. J Immunol 136(7):2348–2357

327. Mosmann TR, Sad S (1996) The expanding universe of T-cell subsets: Th1, Th2 and more. Immunol Today 17(3):138–146

328. Musashi M, Yang YC, Paul SR et al (1991) Direct and synergistic effects of interleukin 11 on murine hemopoiesis in culture. Proc Natl Acad Sci U S A 88(3):765–769

329. Naito K, Tamahashi N, Chiba T et al (1992) The microvasculature of the human bone marrow correlated with the distribution of hematopoietic cells. A computer-assisted three-dimensional reconstruction study. Tohoku J Exp Med 166(4):439–450

330. Naito M (1993) Macrophage heterogeneity in development and differentiation. Arch Histol Cytol 56(4):331–351

331. Ninomiya M, Abe A, Katsumi A et al (2007) Homing, proliferation and survival sites of human leukemia cells in vivo in immunodeficient mice. Leukemia 21(1):136–142

332. Nissen C, Moser Y, Speck B et al (1983) Dexamethasone enhances 'CSA' release and depresses 'BPA' release. Br J Haematol 53(2):301–310

333. Nishi Y, Yoshikawa K, Hiai H et al (1982) Formation of symbiotic complex by microenvironment-dependent mouse leukemias and thymic epithelial reticular cells. J Natl Cancer Inst 69(3):627–637

334. O'Garra A (1989) Interleukins and the immune system 1. Lancet 1(8644):943–947

335. Ohki K, Kohashi O (1994) Laminin promotes proliferation of bone marrow-derived macrophages and macrophage cell lines. Cell Struct Funct 19(2):63–71

336. Okada S, Suda T, Suda J et al (1991) Effects of interleukin 3, interleukin 6, and granulocyte colony-stimulating factor on sorted murine splenic progenitor cells. Exp Hematol 19(1):42–46

337. Otsuka T, Ogo T, Nakano T et al (1994) Expression of the c-kit ligand and interleukin 6 genes in mouse bone marrow stromal cell lines. Stem Cells 12(4):409–415

338. Patchen ML, MacVittie TJ (1985) Stimulated hemopoiesis and enhanced survival following glucan treatment in sublethally and lethally irradiated mice. Int J Immunopharmacol 7(6):923–932

339. Pellegrino TC, Bayer BM (2002) Role of central 5-HT(2) receptors in fluoxetine-induced decreases in T lymphocyte activity. Brain Behav Immun 16(2):87–103

340. Perry MJ, Samuels A, Bird D, Tobias JH (2000) Effects of high-dose estrogen on murine hematopoietic bone marrow precede those on osteogenesis. Am J Physiol Endocrinol Metab 279(5):E1159–1165

341. Pospisil M, Zakopalova I, Netikova J (1972) The effect of hydrocortisone pretreatment upon erythropoietic recovery after a single sublethal x-ray exposure of mice. Folia Biol (Praha) 18(4):284–291

342. Pourtier-Manzanedo A, Didier A, Froidevaux S, Loor F (1995) Lymphotoxicity and myelotoxicity of doxorubicin and SDZ PSC 833 combined chemotherapies for normal mice. Toxicology 99(3):207–217

343. Qiu Y, Peng Y, Wang J (1996) Immunoregulatory role of neurotransmitters. Adv Neuroimmunol 6(3):223–231

344. Rafii S, Mohle R, Shapiro F et al (1997) Regulation of hematopoiesis by microvascular endothelium. Leuk Lymphoma 27(5–6):375–386

345. Ray RJ, Paige CJ, Furlonger C et al (1996) Flt3 ligand supports the differentiation of early B cell progenitors in the presence of interleukin-11 and interleukin-7. Eur J Immunol 26(7): 1504–1510

346. Rich IN, Heit W, Kubanek B (1982) Extrarenal erythropoietin production by macrophages. Blood 60(11):1007–1018

347. Rinehart J, Keville L, Measel J et al (1995) Corticosteroid alteration of carboplatin-induced hematopoietic toxicity in a murine model. Blood 86(12):4493–4499

348. Rutherford MS, Witsell A, Schook LB (1993) Mechanisms generating functionally heterogeneous macrophages: chaos revisited. J Leukoc Biol 53(5):602–618

349. Sakata S, Enoki Y, Ueda M (1992) Relationships between erythropoietin and erythroid colony-stimulating activity in mouse plasma. Zool Sci 9(6):1251

350. Savary CA, Lotzova E (1990) Inhibition of human bone marrow and myeloid progenitors by interleukin 2-activated lymphocytes. Exp Hematol 18(10):1083–1089

351. Schwarzenberger P, Huang W, Ye P et al (2000) Requirement of endogenous stem cell factor and granulocyte-colony-stimulating factor for IL-17-mediated granulopoiesis. J Immunol 164(9):4783–4789

352. Setchenska MS, Bonanou-Tzedaki SA, Arnstein HR (1986) Classification of beta-adrenergic subtypes in immature rabbit bone marrow erythroblasts. Biochem Pharmacol 35(21): 3679–3684

353. Shebalin AI, Frolov NA, Gol'dberg ED et al (2000) Alternative technology of drugs elaboration on the base of velvet deer farming products. The 1st international symposium on Antler Science and Product Technology. Abstracts. Banff Centre, Banff, p 55

354. Shin KH (2000) Immuno-stimulating, anti-stress and antithrombotic activities of unossified pilose antlers. The 1st international symposium on Antler Science and Product Technology. Abstracts. Banff Centre, Banff, p 33

355. Siczkowski M, Andrew T, Amos S, Gordon MY (1993) Hyaluronic acid regulates the function and distribution of sulfated glycosaminoglycans in bone marrow stromal cultures. Exp Hematol 21(1):126–130

356. Sim JS, Sunwoo HH (2000) Antler products and processing technology for the newly emerging functional food market: physico-chemical characteristics of antler products. The 1st international symposium on Antler Science and Product Technology. Abstracts. Banff Centre, Banff, p 34

357. Sonoda Y (1994) Interleukin-4 – a dual regulatory factor in hematopoiesis. Leuk Lymphoma 14(3–4):231–240

358. Stern R (2003) Devising a pathway for hyaluronan catabolism: are we there yet? Glycobiology 13(12):105R–115R

359. Taipale J, Keski-Oja J (1997) Growth factors in the extracellular matrix. FASEB J 11(1):51–59

360. Taneja R, Rameshwar P, Upperman J et al (2000) Effects of hypoxia on granulocytic-monocytic progenitors in rats. Role of bone marrow stroma. Am J Hematol 64(1):20–25

361. Taub DD, Cox GW (1995) Murine Th1 and Th2 cell clones differentially regulate macrophage nitric oxide production. J Leukoc Biol 58(1):80–89

362. Trentin JJ (1976) Hemopoietic inductive microenvironment: stem cells of renewing cell populations. New York, pp 155–164

363. Tsao CW, Lin YS, Cheng JT (1997) Effect of dopamine on immune cell proliferation in mice. Life Sci 61(24):L361–371

364. Turner C, Devitt A, Parker K et al (2003) Macrophage-mediated clearance of cells undergoing caspase-3-independent death. Cell Death Differ 10(3):302–312

365. Udupa KB, Lipschitz DA (1984) Erythropoiesis in the aged mouse: II. Response to stimulation in vitro. J Lab Clin Med 103(4):581–588

366. Verfaillie CM, Catanzarro PM, Li WN (1994) Macrophage inflammatory protein 1 alpha, interleukin 3 and diffusible marrow stromal factors maintain human hematopoietic stem cells for at least eight weeks in vitro. J Exp Med 179(2):643–649

367. Vogel W, Berndt A, Müller A et al (2003) Differential in vivo and in vitro expression of ED-B+ fibronectin in adult human hematopoiesis. Int J Mol Med 12(6):831–837

368. Wajeman-Chao SA, Lancaster SA, Graf LH Jr, Chambers DA (1998) Mechanism of catecholamine-mediated destabilization of messenger RNA encoding Thy-1 protein in T-lineage cells. J Immunol 161(9):4825–4833

369. Walsh RN, Cummins RA (1976) The Open-Field Test: a critical review. Psychol Bull 83(3):482–504

370. Wan Y, Bramson J (2001) Role of dendritic cell-derived cytokines in immune regulation. Curr Pharm Des 7(11):977–992

371. Wilson JG (1997) Adhesive interactions in hemopoiesis. Acta Haematol 97(1–2):6–12

372. Wilson JG, Tavassoli M (1994) Microenvironmental factors involved in the establishment of erythropoiesis in bone marrow. Ann N Y Acad Sci 718:271–283

373. Yang GS, Wang C, Minkin S et al (1991) Hydrocortisone in culture protects the blast cells in acute myeloblastic leukemia from the lethal effects of cytosine arabinoside. J Cell Physiol 148(1):60–67

374. Yang M, Li K, Ng PC et al (2007) Promoting effects of serotonin on hematopoiesis: ex vivo expansion of cord blood CD34+ stem/progenitor cells, proliferation of bone marrow stromal cells, and antiapoptosis. Stem Cells 25(7):1800–1806

375. Yokota T, Meka CS, Kouro T et al (2003) Adiponectin, a fat cell product, influences the earliest lymphocyte precursors in bone marrow cultures by activation of the cyclooxygenase-prostaglandin pathway in stromal cells. J Immunol 171(10):5091–5099

376. Zipori D (1989) Stromal cells from the bone marrow: evidence for a restrictive role in regulation of hemopoiesis. Eur J Haematol 42(3):225–232

377. White C, Yuan X, Schmidt PJ et al (2013) HRG1 is essential for heme transport from the phagolysosome of macrophages during erythrophagocytosis. Cell Metab 17(2):261–270

378. Nishio M, Yoneshiro T, Nakahara M et al (2012) Production of functional classical brown adipocytes from human pluripotent stem cells using specific hemopoietin cocktail without gene transfer. Cell Metab 16(3):394–406

379. Ellis SL, Nilsson SK (2012) The location and cellular composition of the hemopoietic stem cell niche. Cytotherapy 14(2):135–143
380. Gordy C, Pua H, Sempowski GD, He YW (2011) Regulation of steady-state neutrophil homeostasis by macrophages. Blood 117(2):618–629
381. Krstic A, Kocic J, Ilic V et al (2012) Effects of IL-17 on erythroid progenitors growth: involvement of MAPKs and GATA transcription factors. J Biol Regul Homeost Agents 26(4):641–652
382. Koulnis M, Pop R, Porpiglia E et al (2011) Identification and analysis of mouse erythroid progenitors using the CD71/TER119 flow-cytometric assay. J Vis Exp 5(54). pii: 2809. doi: 10.3791/2809.
383. Liu LN, Guo ZW, Zhang Y et al (2012) Polysaccharide extracted from Rheum tanguticum prevents irradiation-induced immune damage in mice. Asian Pac J Cancer Prev 13(4): 1401–1405
384. Miroshnichenko LA, Zhdanov VV, Zyuz'kov GN et al (2010) The mechanisms of hemo-stimulating effects of granulocyte CSF and pantohematogen during cytostatic myelosuppression. Byull Eksp Biol Med 150(12):645–649
385. Dygai AM, Zhdanov VV, Miroshnichenko LA et al (2013) The mechanisms of stimulating effect of glycyramum and D-glucuronic acid on granulocytopoiesis suppressed y 5-fluorouracil. Byull Eksp Biol Med 155(2):170–175
386. Baba J, Watanabe S, Saida Y et al (2012) Depletion of radio-resistant regulatory T cells enhances antitumor immunity during recovery from lymphopenia. Blood 120(12): 2417–2427
387. Stewart FA, Akleyev AV, Hauer-Jensen M (2012) ICRP publication 118: ICRP statement on tissue reactions and early and late effects of radiation in normal tissues and organs – threshold doses for tissue reactions in a radiation protection context. Ann ICRP 41(1–2):1–322